Recent Advances in

Paediatrics
25

Recent Advances in Paediatrics 24
Edited by T.J. David

ISBN 978–1–85315–725–7
ISSN 0–309–0140

Recent Advances in

Paediatrics
25

Edited by

Timothy J. David MB ChB MD PhD FRCP FRCPCH DCH

Professor of Child Health and Paediatrics,
University of Manchester;
Honorary Consultant Paediatrician,
Booth Hall Children's Hospital, Manchester, UK

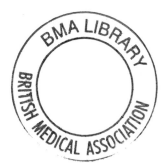

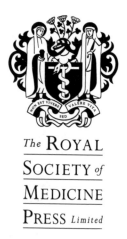

The ROYAL
SOCIETY *of*
MEDICINE
PRESS Limited

© 2009 Royal Society of Medicine Press Ltd
Published by the Royal Society of Medicine Press Ltd
1 Wimpole Street, London W1G 0AE, UK
Tel: +44 (0)20 7290 2921
Fax: +44 (0)20 7290 2929
Email: publishing@rsm.ac.uk
Website: www.rsmpress.co.uk

British Library Cataloguing in Publication Data
A catalogue record for this book is available from the British Library
ISBN 978–1–85315–806–3
ISSN 0–309–0140

Distribution in Europe and Rest of World:

Marston Book Services Ltd
PO Box 269, Abingdon
Oxon OX14 4YN, UK
Tel: +44 (0)1235 465500
Fax: +44 (0)1235 465555
Email: direct.order@marston.co.uk

Distribution in the USA and Canada:

Royal Society of Medicine Press Ltd
c/o BookMasters Inc
30 Amberwood Parkway
Ashland, OH 44805, USA
Tel: +1 800 247 6553/+1 800 266 5564
Fax: +1 419 281 6883
Email: order@bookmasters.com

Distribution in Australia and New Zealand:

Elsevier Australia
30-52 Smidmore Street
Marrikville NSW 2204, Australia
Tel: +61 2 9517 8999
Fax: +61 2 9517 2249
Email: service@elsevier.com.au

Editorial services and typesetting by GM & BA Haddock, Ford, Midlothian, UK
Printed and bound in India by Replika Press Pvt. Ltd.

Contents

Preface

The aim of *Recent Advances in Paediatrics* is to provide a review of important topics and help doctors keep abreast of developments in the subject. The book is intended for the practising clinician, those in specialty training, and doctors preparing for specialty examinations. The book is sold widely in Britain, Europe, North America and Asia, and the contents and authorship are selected with this broad readership in mind. There are 11 chapters, which cover a variety of general paediatric, neonatal and community paediatric areas. As usual, the selection of topics has veered towards those of general rather than special interest.

I am indebted to the authors for their hard work, prompt delivery of manuscripts and patience in dealing with my queries and requests. I would also like to thank Gill and Bruce Haddock of the RSM Press for all their help. Working on a book such as this makes huge inroads into one's spare time, and my special thanks go to my wife and sons for all their support.

Professor Timothy J. David
University of Manchester
Booth Hall Children's Hospital
Manchester M9 7AA, UK
E-mail: tim.david@manchester.ac.uk

Miles Weinberger

1

Cough misdiagnosed as asthma

COUGH AND ITS CAUSES

WHAT IS A COUGH?

A cough involves a forceful expiration that follows an inspiratory gasp and closure of the glottis. A high pressure, as much as 300 mmHg, created by contraction of the diaphragm and accessory muscles of respiration during closure of the glottis is followed a sudden release of the resultant compressed air when the glottis is open. The sudden high flow rate of expired air that then occurs is recognised as a cough. Although a cough can be initiated and suppressed voluntarily, involuntary cough occurs as a result of a complex reflex involving afferent sensory nerve fibres carried to the central nervous system cough centre, following which the vagus, phrenic, and spinal motor nerves carry efferent signals to the larynx, diaphragm, chest and abdominal muscles, and the pelvic floor.

Cough plays an important physiological role in normal airway clearance of excessive mucous and foreign material that enter the airway. Chronic cough is a common, and often challenging, presentation in paediatric patients. It is a symptom of a wide array of underlying disorders.

COUGH AND ASTHMA

Asthma is a disease characterised by hyper-responsiveness of the airways to various stimuli resulting in airway obstruction that is reversible either spontaneously or as a result of treatment. The airway obstruction is from variable components of bronchial smooth muscle spasm and inflammation

Miles Weinberger MD
Professor of Pediatrics, Director, Pediatric Allergy & Pulmonary Division, University of Iowa College of Medicine, 200 Hawkins Drive, Iowa City, IA 52242, USA
E-mail: miles-weinberger@uiowa.edu

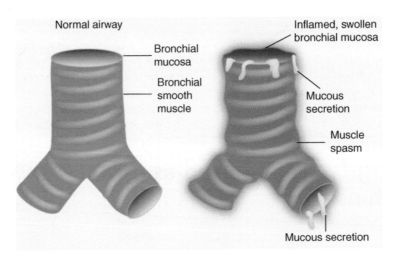

Fig. 1 Artist's rendition of the two components of airway obstruction in asthma: bronchospasm and inflammation with mucosal oedema and mucous secretions.

that result in oedema of the respiratory mucosa and mucous secretions (Fig. 1). Since cough is a natural response to clear mucous from the airway, cough is a common symptom of asthma.

In a survey of children with asthma at the University of Iowa Pediatric Allergy & Pulmonary Clinic, cough was as frequent a symptom as wheeze among children with clinical asthma, with cough and wheeze typically occurring concomitantly. However, there was a minority of patients in whom cough was the only prominent symptom. Published descriptions of such patients, sometimes referred to as cough variant asthma, were described over 30 years ago for adults[1] and children.[2,3]

Since cough is a common presenting symptom of children for whom medical care is sought, and asthma is the most common chronic disease of children, the presence of cough without an obvious alternative diagnosis certainly warrants including asthma in the differential diagnosis. However, despite the high prevalence of asthma and its common presentation as cough, there are many causes of cough other than asthma, some of which are all too frequently misdiagnosed as asthma as a consequence of not considering the range of less common disorders for which cough is a prominent symptom.

What is asthma?

In considering the aetiology of cough, it is essential to consider the definition of asthma in order to assess if the coughing patient's clinical course is consistent with asthma. Asthma is a disease characterised by hyper-responsiveness of the airways to various stimuli resulting in airway obstruction that is reversible, either spontaneously or as a result of treatment. The airway obstruction is from variable components of bronchial smooth muscle spasm and inflammation that result in oedema of the respiratory mucosa and mucous secretions. The bronchial smooth muscle spasm is highly responsive to an inhaled β_2-adrenergic agonist bronchodilator, and the inflammation is highly responsive to a short course of high-dose oral corticosteroids.

When is it not asthma?

Asthma is diagnosed clinically and is suspected when there is recurrent or chronic cough, wheezing, or dyspnoea. Since the presence of cough alone can occur with asthma but is responsive to a short course of high-dose oral corticosteroid,[4] the lack of response to a trial of oral corticosteroid identifies patients whose symptoms must be considered as being from some cause other than asthma. While dose-response data for oral corticosteroids are limited, empirically 2 mg/kg/dose of prednisolone or equivalent administered twice daily to a maximum of 40 mg twice daily (reducing to once daily in the morning if insomnia or irritability becomes problematic) provides a sufficient dose for a diagnostic therapeutic trial. Failure to observe substantial improvement within 5–7 days with complete relief of signs and symptoms of asthma argues against asthma as the aetiology, assuming, of course, that the patient has actually taken the prescribed medication.

COUGH THAT IS NOT ASTHMA

Asthma is the most common cause of chronic or recurrent inflammatory airway disease and a major cause of cough. While there are causes of cough that are unlikely to be confused with asthma, there are several referred to the Pediatric Allergy and Pulmonary Clinic at the Children's Hospital of Iowa that have been confused with asthma with the result being over-diagnosis of asthma with consequent inappropriate treatment.[5]

Whooping cough

Infection from *Bordetella pertussis*, known in the past as the 100-day cough, causes a prolonged period of cough, and we have seen several cases where the primary care physician prescribed anti-asthmatic medication because pertussis was not adequately considered. While the cough is characteristically

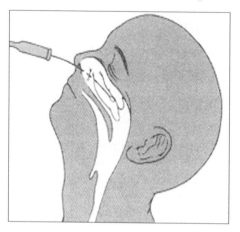

Fig. 2 Pertussis should be considered for any child with a prolonged period of cough in the absence of a prior history. A flexible wire with a cotton tip is inserted in a nare and left in the posterior nasopharynx for 30 s before being withdrawn, appropriately saved as instructed by the laboratory, and sent for polymerase chain reaction (PCR) detection of pertussis. This is far more sensitive than culture. When performed early in the course of pertussis infection, appropriate preventative measures can be provided to all contacts and, thereby, minimisation of the spread.

spasmodic and associated with post-tussive gagging or emesis, the classical clinical symptoms are often not present in an immunised population. In fact, evidence for *B. pertussis* infection has been identified in 10–30% of immunised children and adults with persistent cough for 2 or more weeks in the absence of a prior history consistent with an underlying disorder.[6–10] Establishing the diagnosis is important to prevent spread to contacts, especially to young infants who are the greatest risk for hospitalisation and fatality from this infection. Diagnosis is most readily made by polymerase chain reaction (PCR) from a properly collected nasal swab to detect pertussis antigen (Fig. 2).

Cystic fibrosis

Cystic fibrosis is the second most common chronic inflammatory airway disease, at least among Caucasians. It occurs in about 1 in 2500 live births in populations of Northern European descent with variable lesser incidence in other ethnic groups and races. Although the mechanisms of airway inflammation are different in these two diseases, both cause airway obstruction, cough, wheezing, and dyspnoea with persistent cough often a prominent symptom.

It has not been unusual at cystic fibrosis centres to encounter delays in diagnosis because of the presumption that persistent cough in a patient was from asthma. This is particularly true for those who are not pancreatic insufficient, as is seen in about 15% of patients with cystic fibrosis. There is considerable variability in the extent to which the mutations of the cystic fibrosis transmembrane regulator gene, now numbering more than 1500, alter the chloride channel and result in clinical manifestations.[11] Consequently, some do not present with respiratory symptoms until adolescence or even as adults.[12] Some degree of bronchodilator response may even be present although the physiology of the airway responsiveness differs from that in asthma.[13] In addition, asthma can co-exist with cystic fibrosis, probably occurring in children with cystic fibrosis as frequently as in the rest of the population.

The absence of the classical clinical presentation of malabsorption and the variable severity and progression of the airway disease of cystic fibrosis are frequent causes for the delay in diagnosis. While that will likely be largely overcome with the current trend towards universal newborn screening, some cystic fibrosis variants may slip through the newborn screening process and continue to be misdiagnosed as asthma if clinicians are not sufficiently critical in assessing asthma as a diagnosis in children with persistent cough.

Cystic fibrosis should be suspected when symptoms and signs of airway inflammatory disease persist despite a short course of high-dose systemic corticosteroid. The diagnosis of cystic fibrosis is most reliably made by performing a sweat chloride measurement using the classical quantitative pilocarpine iontophoresis method. The various commercial methods utilising assessment by the conductivity of sweat are unreliable, having both false-positive and false-negative results.[14] For the test to be valid, duplicate collections of at least 75 mg are required for the filter paper discs or gauze pads with duplicate 15 µl samples being sufficient with the Macroduct collection coil.[15] Measurement of 60 meq/l chloride with substantial agreement in duplicate samples is generally diagnostic of cystic fibrosis. Sweat chloride concentrations of less than 40 meq/l are generally re-assuring that cystic fibrosis is not the cause of the patient's airway inflammatory disease. Levels of 40–60 meq/l (over 30 meq/l for infants) are considered sufficiently suspicious that genetic analysis should be performed for the presence of two mutations of the cystic fibrosis transmembrane regulator gene.[16] About 1% of patients with some of the less common mutations of cystic fibrosis do not have elevated sweat chloride levels.[11,17] While rare, awareness of these exceptional cases with normal sweat chloride levels permits specific treatment rather than fruitless use of anti-asthmatic medications that only frustrate the patient and the physician.

Primary ciliary dyskinesia

This disorder is rare, with an estimated prevalence of about 1 in 50,000, and should be considered only when a persistent cough is present virtually from birth, generally in association with chronic otitis media.[18] A degree of neonatal respiratory distress is commonly present.[19] It includes a variety of abnormalities in airway ciliary structure and/or function that result in the absence of normal mucociliary clearance, an important innate host-defence mechanism for the lungs. A continuous flow of the mucous layer of the respiratory mucosa is normally maintained by the co-ordinated rhythmic beating of ciliated respiratory epithelial cells. The absence of the co-ordinated ciliary movement results in pooling of mucous in the airway associated with low-grade chronic infection. Cough and slowly progressing bronchiectasis result from this defect. Half will have situs inversus totalis where it is known as Kartagener's syndrome. As with cystic fibrosis, primary ciliary dyskinesia will not respond to usual anti-asthmatic medications, and delayed diagnosis results in permanently damaged airways.

The diagnosis should be highly suspect in the presence of situs inversus totalis, with primary ciliary dysfunction present in about 30% of those with that anatomical disorder. The definitive diagnosis can be difficult in the absence of that anatomical abnormality.[20] The cough is typically present since birth on a daily basis without the fluctuating course of asthma. Chronic otitis media is another characteristic feature of the disorder. The classical means of diagnosis has been examination of ciliary structure by electron microscopy. However, this is fraught with errors in interpretation. Examination of co-ordinated ciliary movement from a nasal or tracheal epithelial sample by light or phase-contrast microscopy is a more practical means for an initial evaluation.

Tracheomalacia and bronchomalacia

Inadequate rigidity of the tracheal or mainstem bronchial cartilage results in tracheal collapse which causes cough by at least two mechanisms. Collapse of the trachea or mainstem bronchi during increased intrathoracic pressure (as in vigorous exhalation or coughing) can cause the anterior and posterior walls to come into contact resulting in an irritable focus that stimulates further cough. Additionally, when secretions are present in the airway, the airway collapse during expiration prevents normal airway clearance. The secretions then act as a continued stimulus for a non-productive cough.

While tracheomalacia (Fig. 3) and bronchomalacia (Fig. 4) can be troublesome in the infant, some cases do not cause problems until later in childhood.[21] In unusually severe cases of intractable cough from

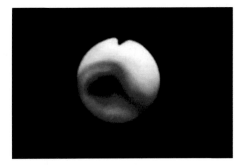

Fig. 3 Tracheomalacia, a softening of the tracheal rings that provide a degree of rigidity to the airway, occurs from either a defect in the cartilage itself or from external compression by the great vessels. The innominate artery (brachiocephalic trunk) crosses over the lower third of the trachea where a pulsating bulge can often be seen on bronchoscopy. This is a common location for tracheomalacia as in this picture. Persistent cough occurs when the repeated contact of the anterior and posterior walls of the trachea causes a focus of irritation with a consequent harsh barking cough characteristic of a tracheal cough. Cough may also occur because of inefficient clearing of secretions that results from the collapse of the airway when intrathoracic pressure is increased during coughing.

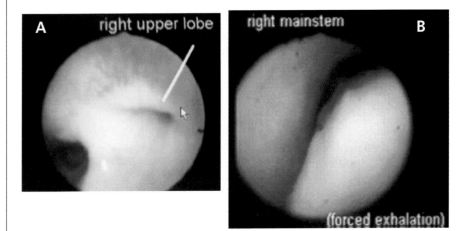

Fig. 4 Bronchomalacia of the right upper lobe (A) and of the right mainstem (B). Depending on the degree of obstruction caused by the malacia, either cough or expiratory monophonic wheezing may be heard. Obstruction occurs on expiration with positive intrathoracic pressure during expiration while negative intrathoracic pressure during inspiration opens the airway. Complete airway obstruction during expiration can result in lobar emphysema from persistent hyperinflation of the lobe distal to the malacia. Decreased clearing of secretions distal to the malacia may result in purulent bacterial bronchitis.

tracheomalacia, surgical aortopexy is needed.[22] This involves placing a suture through the adventitial lining of the aortic arch and the periostium of the sternum to pull the arch forward. Since there is connective tissue between the anterior tracheal wall and the aortic arch, this procedure essentially stents the anterior wall of the trachea thereby maintaining a more patent tracheal lumen and preventing the repeated irritating contact of the anterior and posterior walls of the vessel.

Chronic purulent (bacterial) bronchitis

This is an entity not well appreciated and only infrequently described.[23,24] While chronic bacterial bronchitis is certainly a characteristic of cystic fibrosis, there are young children with no identifiable abnormalities in immunity or other underlying disease who have prolonged periods of cough with neutrophilia and bacteria in their lower airways demonstrable by broncho-alveolar lavage. Some, but not all, have bronchomalacia that may be contributing both to cough and to retaining secretions in the lower airway which predisposes the child to secondary infection (Fig. 4).

The bacteria identified are most commonly the same as those commonly associated with otitis media – *Haemophilus* spp., *Moraxella catarrhalis* and, occasionally, *Streptococcus pneumoniae.*[23,24] While responsive to appropriate antibiotics, some will require repeated courses or even maintenance prophylactic antibiotics for an extended period. Resolution with age is common in the absence of an additional underlying innate or acquired host defence disorder. Diagnosis requires flexible bronchoscopy and broncho-alveolar lavage with cell count and differential for evidence of significant neutrophilia (greater than 10% of total while cell count) and quantitative culture of lavage fluid.

Habit cough syndrome

This is a troublesome disorder commonly treated as asthma that often causes a great deal of morbidity and ineffective treatment and yet is readily rapidly curable with suggestion therapy, a simple behavioural technique.[25] The classical presentation of the habit cough syndrome is that of a harsh, barking, repetitive cough occurring several times per minute for hours on end (video available at <http://www.mastersofpediatrics.com/cme/cme2006/lecture38_1.asp>). It is extremely irritating to those in the presence of the individual suffering from this disorder. Characteristic of the habit cough syndrome is the complete absence of cough once the patient is asleep. Frequently subjected to multiple diagnostic tests and therapy with anti-asthmatic medications, this disorder should be readily diagnosed by the characteristic barking nature of the cough, its repetitive pattern, and absence once the patient is asleep.

This syndrome is sometimes misinterpreted as a tic. However, the so-called cough-tic syndrome will involve more vocalisation characteristic of Tourette's syndrome and does not resemble the typical tracheal sounding cough of the habit cough syndrome. In considering treatment and discussing the issue with the family, it is important not to refer to this as a psychogenic cough, since that is likely to affect the relationship with the therapist adversely, who will subsequently need the patient's rapport to utilise suggestion therapy effectively. Moreover, other psychosomatic or psychological problems appear to be uncommon in these children and adolescents. Although Anbar and Hall[26] reported a high incidence of abdominal pain and irritable bowel syndrome in many of the children with habit cough syndrome, a standardised psychological questionnaire administered to our patients subsequent to successful treatment of the habit cough with suggestion therapy found no other evidence for somatisation. However, the questionnaire revealed some tendency to score high, but not pathologically so, on an obsessive-compulsive scale.[25] Perhaps related to this personality characteristic is our observation that most of these patients were academically high achievers.

Table 1 The major elements of the suggestion therapy session for the habit cough syndrome

- Expressing confidence, communicated verbally and behaviourally, that the therapist will be able to show the patient how to stop the cough

- Explaining the cough as a vicious cycle of an initial irritant, now gone, that had set up a pattern of coughing which caused irritation and further symptoms

- Encouraging the suppression of cough in order to break the cycle. The therapist closely observes for the initiation of the muscular movement preceding coughing and immediately exhorts the patient to hold the cough back, emphasising that each second the cough is delayed makes further inhibition of cough easier

- An alternative behaviour to coughing is offered in the form of inhaling a gene-rated mist or sipping body-temperature water with encouragement to inhale the mist or sip the water every time they begin to feel the urge to cough

- Repeating expressions of confidence that the patient was developing the ability to resist the urge to cough

- When some ability to suppress cough is observed (usually after about 10 min), asking in a rhetorical manner if they are beginning to feel that they can resist the urge to cough, e.g. 'You're beginning to feel that you can resist the urge to cough, aren't you?'

- Discontinuing the session when the patient can repeatedly answer positively to the question: 'Do you feel that you can now resist the urge to cough on your own?' This question is only asked after the patient has gone 5 min without coughing

If not treated with appropriate behavioural intervention, symptoms can continue for months and years as was demonstrated in a follow-up of diagnoses of habit cough syndrome made at the Mayo Clinic.[27] Treatment with suggestion therapy has provided a sustained cure by the use of various techniques. In 1966, Berman[28] described six patients with this disorder who were successfully treated with therapy that 'relied solely on the art of suggestion'. Another report[29] utilised a tightly wrapped bedsheet around the chest combined with the suggestion that this would stop the coughing. Teaching self-hypnosis to stop the cough has been described with a high success rate using a technique that appears to be essentially a variation of suggestion therapy.[26] We have used a technique that generally results in complete cessation of symptoms within 15 min (Table 1).[25,30]

Other rare causes of chronic cough misdiagnosed as asthma

While unlikely to be frequently encountered, awareness of these entities can encourage further investigation when the pattern of symptoms and response to treatment is not consistent with asthma. A uvula that was in contact with the epiglottis was the cause of a long-standing cough in a 4-year-old boy treated unsuccessfully for asthma.[31] This could be visualised only during flexible fibre-optic bronchoscopy while he was lying on his back. The child related that he coughed because he felt something in the back of his throat. His cough was cured with uvulectomy (Fig. 5). Tonsils impinging on the uvula of a 3-year-old girl were seen on bronchoscopy with chronic cough initially treated as asthma (Fig. 6). Tonsillectomy cured the cough in that patient and another with similar findings.

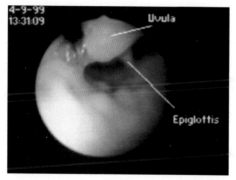

Fig. 5 The uvula making contact with the epiglottis caused a troublesome cough in this 4-year-old boy treated unsuccessfully for asthma who was able to relate that he coughed because he felt something in the back of his throat. Uvulectomy cured his cough.[31]

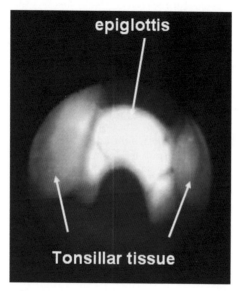

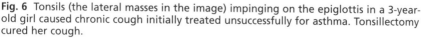

Fig. 6 Tonsils (the lateral masses in the image) impinging on the epiglottis in a 3-year-old girl caused chronic cough initially treated unsuccessfully for asthma. Tonsillectomy cured her cough.

Controversial causes of cough

Cough is often attributed to gastro-oesophageal reflux or post-nasal drip, termed by some as upper airway cough syndrome.[32] However, these diagnoses are infrequently supported by objective evidence. When broncho-alveolar lavage was performed as part of a diagnostic study for protracted cough in children, neither the so-called upper airway cough syndrome nor gastro-oesophageal reflux were common diagnoses.[24] Post-nasal mucus may certainly be visualised in the posterior oral pharynx but there is considerable scepticism that this is a cause of true cough rather than just throat clearing for some.[33,34] Similarly, since gastro-oesophageal reflux can result from coughing,[35] there is an on-going debate with inconclusive evidence regarding this chicken-and-egg question.[36]

Key points for clinical practice

- Recurring or chronic cough is a common presenting problem to physicians.

- Asthma will generally be the most common cause of recurrent or chronic cough.

- The most efficient means of diagnosing asthma is a short course of an oral corticosteroid at a dose of 2 mg/kg/dose of prednisolone or equivalent administered twice daily. Failure of complete cessation of cough within 7–10 days indicates a cause other than asthma. If asthma is confirmed, further evaluation can determine an appropriate treatment plan to manage recurrent or chronic cough from this common disorder.

- If no prior history of a persistent cough, consider whooping cough, even in previously immunised children and adults. A nasopharyngeal swab sent for detection of *Bordetella pertussis* antigen by polymerase chain reaction (PCR).

- Cystic fibrosis should be considered if cough does not respond to the diagnostic test with an oral corticosteroid. Evaluation with a sweat chloride test at a cystic fibrosis centre provides assurance that a proper sweat chloride collection and analysis is performed. If suspicion persists despite normal sweat chloride values, genetic testing for mutations can identify the rare mutations associated with normal sweat chloride values despite the lung disease of cystic fibrosis.

- If present since birth, especially if accompanied by chronic otitis media, refer to a centre with the capability of diagnosing primary ciliary dysfunction.

- Once cough is determined to be neither asthma nor pertussis and is present nocturnally once asleep, consider tracheomalacia, bronchomalacia, or chronic purulent bronchitis by referring to a centre that can perform flexible fibre-optic bronchoscopy with conscious sedation. Rigid bronchoscopy under general anaesthesia will frequently miss dynamic abnormalities of the airway. Bronchoscopic data should include cell count and differential and quantitative culture.

- Harsh barking repetitive cough in a school-age child or adolescent that is not present once asleep is the typical presentation for the habit cough syndrome. Treatment with suggestion therapy is highly successful. Failure to treat with suggestion therapy is associated with continued prolonged morbidity.

- Other rare causes of cough from anatomical irritation of the epiglottis by an uvula or tonsils can be identified by flexible fibre-optic bronchoscopy.

- The common practice of attributing chronic cough to gastro-oesophageal reflux or post-nasal drainage is not supported by evidence. Pursuing those diagnoses is, therefore, generally not justified.

References

1. Corrao WM, Braman SS, Irwin RS. Chronic cough as the sole presenting manifestation of bronchial asthma. *N Engl J Med* 1979; **300**: 633–637.
2. Hannaway PJ, Hopper DK. Cough variant asthma in children. *JAMA* 1982; **247**: 206–208.
3. Yahav Y, Katznelson D, Benzaray S. Persistent cough – a *forme-fruste* of asthma. *Eur J Respir Dis* 1982; **63**: 43–46.
4. Doan T, Patterson R, Greenberger PA. Cough variant asthma: usefulness of a diagnostic-therapeutic trial with prednisone. *Ann Allergy* 1992; **69**: 505–509.
5. Thomson F, Masters IB, Chang AB. Persistent cough in children and the overuse of medications. *J Paediatr Child Health* 2002; **38**: 578–581.
6. Mink CM, Cherry JD, Christenson P *et al*. A search for *Bordetella pertussis* infection in university students. *Clin Infect Dis* 1992; **14**: 464–471.
7. Wright SW, Edwards KM, Decker MD, Zeldin MH. Pertussis infection in adults with persistent cough. *JAMA* 1995; **273**: 1044–1046.
8. Nennig ME, Shinefield HR, Edwards KM, Black SB, Fireman BH. Prevalence and incidence of adult pertussis in an urban population. *JAMA* 1996; **275**: 1672–1674.
9. Craig AS, Wright SW, Edwards KM *et al*. Outbreak of pertussis on a college campus. *Am J Med* 2007; **120**: 364–368.
10. Harnden A, Grant C, Harrison T *et al*. Whooping cough in school age children with persistent cough: prospective cohort study in primary care. *BMJ* 2006; **333**: 174–177.
11. Wilschanski M, Dupuis A, Ellis L *et al*. Mutations in the cystic fibrosis transmembrane regulator gene and *in vivo* transepithelial potentials. *Am J Respir Crit Care Med* 2006; **174**: 787–794.
12. Gilljam M, Ellis L, Corey M, Zielenski J, Durie P, Tullis DE. Clinical manifestations of cystic fibrosis among patients with diagnosis in adulthood. *Chest* 2004; **126**: 1215–1224.
13. Weinberger M. Airways reactivity in patients with CF. *Clin Rev Allergy Immunol* 2002; **23**: 77–85.
14. Denning CR, Huang NN, Cuasay LR *et al*. Cooperative study comparing three methods of performing sweat tests to diagnose cystic fibrosis. *Pediatrics* 1980; **66**: 752–757.
15. National Committee for Clinical Laboratory Standards. *Sweat testing: sample collection and quantitative analysis-approved guideline* [document C34-A]. Wayne, PA: NCCLS, 1994 [Address: 940 W. Valley Rd., Suite 1400, Wayne, PA 19087, USA].
16. Cystic Fibrosis Mutation Database. <http://www.genet.sickkids.on.ca/cftr/StatisticsPage.html>.
17. Highsmith WE, Burch LH, Zhou Z *et al*. A novel mutation in the cystic fibrosis gene in patients with pulmonary disease but normal sweat chloride concentrations, *N Engl J Med* 1994; **331**: 974–980.
18. Leigh MW. Primary ciliary dyskinesia. In: Chernick V, Boat TF, Wilmott RW, Bush A. (eds) *Kendig's Disorders of the Respiratory Tract in Children*, 7th edn. Philadelphia, PA: Saunders Elsevier, 2006; 902–909.
19. Ferkol T, Leigh M. Primary ciliary dyskinesia and newborn respiratory distress. *Semin Perinatol* 2006; **30**: 335–340.
20. Bush A, Chodhari R, Collins N *et al*. Primary ciliary dyskinesia: current state of the art. *Arch Dis Child* 2007; **92**: 1136–1140.
21. Wood RE. Localized tracheomalacia or bronchomalacia in children with intractable cough. *J Pediatr* 1990; **116**: 404–406.
22. Weber TR, Keller MS, Fiore A. Aortic suspension (aortopexy) for severe tracheomalacia in infants and children. *Am J Surg* 2002; **184**: 573–577.
23. Saito J, Harris WT, Gelfond J *et al*. Physiologic, bronchoscopic, and bronchoalveolar lavage fluid findings in young children with recurrent wheeze and cough. *Pediatr Pulmonol* 2006; **41**: 709–719.
24. Marchant JM, Masters IB, Taylor SM *et al*. Evaluation and outcome of young children with chronic cough. *Chest* 2006; **129**: 1132–1141.
25. Lokshin B, Lindgren S, Weinberger M, Koviach J. Outcome of habit cough in children treated with a brief session of suggestion therapy. *Ann Allergy* 1991; **67**: 579–582.
26. Anbar RD, Hall HR. Childhood habit cough treated with self-hypnosis. *J Pediatr* 2004; **144**: 213–217.

27. Rojas AR, Sachs MI, Yunginger JW, O'Connell EJ. Childhood involuntary cough syndrome: a long-term follow-up study. *Ann Allergy* 1991; **66**: 106.
28. Berman BA. Habit cough in adolescent children. *Ann Allergy* 1966; **24**: 43–46.
29. Cohlan SQ, Stone SM. The cough and the bedsheet. *Pediatrics* 1984; **74**: 11–15.
30. Lokshin B, Weinberger M. The habit cough syndrome: a review. *Am J Asthma Allergy Pediatr* 1993; **7**: 11–15.
31. Najada A, Weinberger M. Unusual cause of chronic cough in a four-year-old cured by uvulectomy. *Pediatr Pulmonol* 2002; **34**: 144–146.
32. Pratter MR, Brightling CE, Boulet LP, Irwin RS. An empiric integrative approach to the management of cough: ACCP evidence-based clinical practice guidelines. *Chest* 2006; **129**: 222S–231S.
33. Morice AH. Post-nasal drip syndrome – a symptom to be sniffed at? *Pulmon Pharmacol Ther* 2004; **17**: 343–345.
34. Kemp A. Does post-nasal drip cause cough in childhood? *Paediatr Resp Rev* 2006; **7**: 31–35.
35. Weinberger M. Gastroesophageal reflux is not a significant cause of lung disease in children. *Pediatr Pulmonol* 2004; **Suppl 26**: 194–196.
36. Chang AB, Lasserson TJ, Gaffney J, Connor FL, Garske LA. Gastro-oesophageal reflux treatment for prolonged non-specific cough in children and adults. Cochrane Database Syst Rev 2006; (4): CD004823.

Joseph J. Zorc

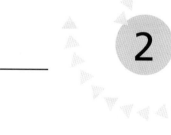

2

Diagnosis and management of bronchiolitis

Bronchiolitis is a clinical syndrome caused by lower respiratory tract infection that occurs commonly in infants and toddlers. The aetiology of bronchiolitis is usually a viral infection, most frequently respiratory syncytial virus, which circulates in annual epidemics during the winter months and infects most children by their second birthday. Bronchiolitis has received increasing attention in recent years due to high rates of hospitalisation and research showing wide variability in diagnostic testing and therapy without a clear relation to outcomes. This controversy has led to systematic reviews of the literature, clinical practice guidelines published by professional groups, and several large multicentre clinical trials. This review will focus on recent additions to the literature on bronchiolitis with emphasis on practical management for clinicians.

CLINICAL EPIDEMIOLOGY

The typical clinical presentation of bronchiolitis is an infant presenting with troubled breathing, cough, or other signs of respiratory distress that develop in the days following the onset of an upper respiratory infection. Physical examination findings include evidence of respiratory distress (such as tachypnoea) and use of accessory muscles; chest examination may show wheezing and diffuse rales. Of note, the definition of bronchiolitis varies somewhat internationally, and this should be kept in mind when interpreting research studies. In the UK, the term bronchiolitis tends to be limited to infants, whereas in North America it may be used more broadly in children up

Joseph J. Zorc MD
Associate Professor of Pediatrics at the University of Pennsylvania School of Medicine and Attending Physician, Division of Emergency Medicine (AS01), The Children's Hospital of Philadelphia, 34th Street and Civic Center Boulevard, Philadelphia, PA 19104-4399, USA
E-mail: zorc@email.chop.edu

to 2 years of age presenting with viral-induced wheeze.[1] More than one in three children will develop bronchiolitis during the first 2 years of life.[2] Of these, about one in ten (approximately 3% of all infants in the US) will be hospitalised, up from about 1% in the 1970s.[3] Although hospitalisations appear to have increased, mortality from bronchiolitis is reported to be low and unchanged over recent decades. Data from the US suggest an infant death rate from bronchiolitis of 2.2 per 100,000 live births.[3,4]

The list of infectious agents that cause bronchiolitis is varied and continues to grow. Respiratory syncytial virus accounts for about 60–70% of bronchiolitis cases.[5,6] Transmission of respiratory syncytial virus occurs from large particle aerosols or, importantly for medical personnel, by direct contact with secretions which remain contagious on skin or surfaces for hours. Re-infection with respiratory syncytial virus leading to upper respiratory infection in adults is common and poses another challenge for prevention of nosocomial infection. Other common viral causes of bronchiolitis include rhinovirus, metapneumovirus, influenza, adenovirus, and parainfluenza. Rhinovirus is a more common aetiology of bronchiolitis after 6 months of age and is associated with higher rates of atopy and a greater risk of later asthma.[7] Metapneumovirus is a recently discovered paramyxovirus similar to respiratory syncytial virus. Examination of samples banked from older studies suggests that it is not actually a new agent and accounts for about 5–15% of bronchiolitis cases.[8] New information is emerging about metapneumovirus, but currently it appears to have a similar clinical course to respiratory syncytial virus.

Examination of the lower airway of a bronchiolitic child shows necrosis and sloughing of epithelial cells with prominent oedema, mucus and infiltration of inflammatory cells. The difficulty that an infant experiences in clearing these products from the airway can lead to some of the hallmark clinical findings of bronchiolitis: (i) variability, as mucus and other products move through the respiratory tract and change findings on examination; (ii) hypoxaemia, due to atelectasis from airway obstruction; and (iii) a prolonged recovery, as normal ciliated epithelial cells require weeks to re-populate the airway. Bronchospasm is also a part of the pathophysiology of bronchiolitis, although its importance and responsiveness to treatment is controversial.

DIAGNOSIS AND LABORATORY TESTING

Diagnosis of bronchiolitis depends primarily on the history and physical examination. A typical case, as defined in a recent research study attempting to reduce the need for further testing, is a previously healthy child, 2–23 months of age, presenting with coryza, cough, and physical findings of respiratory distress and wheezing.[9] Despite this common and recognisable clinical presentation, diagnostic uncertainty among clinicians is demonstrated by studies showing wide variability in the use of laboratory tests internationally.[10,11] For example, one study of 30 US children's hospitals found hospital rates of chest radiography ranging from 38% to 89% and respiratory syncytial virus testing from 26% to 92% among patients admitted for bronchiolitis. These tests may be ordered for a variety of reasons, including: to support a clinical diagnosis of viral bronchiolitis, to rule out other concomitant conditions, to assess current severity, or to predict outcomes that may assist with management decisions. However, when examined critically, systematic reviews of the literature have found little evidence to support routine use of tests for any of these indications in typical presentations of bronchiolitis.[12] In addition, recent evidence has identified potential negative effects of testing, such as increased use of antibiotics after chest radiography.[9] These findings are supported by prospective efforts which have demonstrated success at reducing testing while improving outcomes and reducing costs.[13]

VIRAL TESTING

There are a variety of tests available to diagnose respiratory syncytial virus and other viruses that cause bronchiolitis. Rapid antigen tests are widely available and have generally good sensitivity and specificity when performed on appropriately collected specimens.[14] However, it is important to recognise that the positive predictive value (probability of true respiratory syncytial virus infection given a positive rapid test) of tests varies widely depending on the pre-test probability, and they are much less accurate in times of low prevalence. For example, if a rapid respiratory syncytial virus test with 90% sensitivity and specificity is positive for a wheezing infant at a time of peak viral activity when the pre-test probability is 70%, the likelihood that the test represents true infection is 95%; the same positive result performed during the summer months, when the pre-test probability is 10%, would have a 50% chance of being a false positive. Newer, polymerase chain reaction (PCR)-based tests have high sensitivity and now represent the gold standard for diagnosis of infection. Given that respiratory syncytial virus tests are most useful when respiratory syncytial virus is most prevalent, one may question the benefit of routine testing (especially at times of seasonally reduced prevalence in the warmer months), and systematic reviews of the literature suggest they rarely alter management decisions.[12] One potential role for respiratory syncytial virus testing includes use for cohorting purposes in tertiary care centres, which has been shown to reduce nosocomial infections.[15] However, cohorting by presence of viral symptoms rather than specific test results may be an effective alternative option given the wide variety of potential viral infections known to cause bronchiolitis.[13]

Another specific scenario where viral tests have been evaluated is the young infant with bronchiolitis and fever where a work-up for bacterial infection is being considered. A multicentre study of 1248 infants under 2 months of age found a significantly lower prevalence of serious bacterial infection among respiratory syncytial virus-positive (7.0%) compared to respiratory syncytial virus-negative (12.5%) infants.[16] Most of the bacterial infections among respiratory syncytial virus-positive infants were urinary tract infections (5.4% prevalence) with no cases of bacterial meningitis. However, it is important to keep in mind that, due to the continued shedding of respiratory syncytial virus for weeks, a positive test from a past infection can accompany a subsequent bacterial infection. Infants with a clinical picture of bronchiolitis had a similarly low prevalence of bacterial infection to respiratory syncytial virus-positive infants (7.1% with no cases of bacteraemia or meningitis), highlighting the value of clinical assessment as opposed to viral testing. Studies of older infants with bronchiolitis have found very low rates of concomitant serious bacterial infection.[2]

CHEST RADIOGRAPHY

Chest radiographs are commonly obtained in infants with bronchiolitis; a study of 30 large US children's hospitals found a rate of 72%.[10] Recent studies have clarified the limited benefit and potential harms of this practice. Schuh *et al.*[9] prospectively enrolled 265 previously healthy children aged 2–23 months with a first episode of wheezing who met pre-defined criteria for typical bronchiolitis including presence of coryza, cough, and a non-toxic appearance. All of the infants had a chest radiograph obtained and only two (0.75%) were inconsistent with bronchiolitis (one with an incidentally discovered atrial septal defect and one with a pneumonia that improved without antibiotic treatment), neither of which led to a change in acute management. Certainly, other diagnoses can present with symptoms similar to bronchiolitis and should be considered in the differential diagnosis (Table 1). However, these results suggest that, in typical cases, the likelihood of another cause is very low, and routine radiography has little benefit. When a radiograph is obtained, the presence of atelectasis or consolidation has been shown to correlate with an increased risk of progression to severe disease; however, it is unclear that this would influence management in most situations.[17,18] The flip side of routine radiography was also demonstrated by the Schuh *et al.*[9] study, as the proportion of physicians planning to prescribe antibiotics increased after reviewing the images. The potential that non-specific findings on radiographs lead to unnecessary treatment with antibiotics has also been demonstrated in a clinical trial across a broader age-range of children.[19] Given these findings, the practice of obtaining a routine radiograph has little support and has successfully been reduced at some institutions while improving overall outcomes.[13]

Table 1 Differential diagnosis for a wheezing infant

• Viral bronchiolitis
• Other pulmonary infections (e.g. pneumonia, *Mycoplasma* spp., *Chlamydia* spp., tuberculosis)
• Laryngotracheomalacia
• Foreign body – oesophageal or aspirated
• Gastro-oesophageal reflux
• Congestive heart failure
• Vascular ring
• Allergic reaction
• Cystic fibrosis
• Mediastinal mass
• Bronchogenic cyst
• Tracheo-oesphageal fistula

ASSESSMENT AND PREDICTION

A primary concern for a clinician assessing a child with bronchiolitis is estimating the risk that the child will progress to severe disease. The clinical course of bronchiolitis is characterised by several sources of temporal variability: minute-to-minute variability in respiratory status due to mucus plugging and other changes in the infant's status, and a more broad progression through the stages of viral infection and recovery. Infants often worsen for 3–5 days and then have a gradual improvement, which can be prolonged, with some not returning to baseline for weeks (39% at 14 days and 9% at 28 days in one study).[20] A few research studies have attempted to predict progression of disease, but have defined it in various ways. One group of studies sought to predict need for hospitalisation in out-patients (Table 2).[17,21,22] Other

Table 2 Selected risk factors for outcomes of bronchiolitis in three prospective studies of out-patients

Risk factors	Outcome		
	Severe disease* Shaw et al.[17]	Hospitalisation Mansbach et al.[22]	Hospitalisation Voets et al.[21]
Age			
< 2 months		4.5/0.78	
< 3 months	2.2/0.75		
< 6 months			2.2/0.53
Prematurity			
< 34 weeks	5.4/0.77		
< 35 weeks		1.5/0.96	
Ill appearance	3.2/0.32		
Oxygen saturation			
< 94%		5.4/0.77	
< 95%	16/0.69		5.2/0.37
Respiratory rate			
> 45			3.8/0.39
≥ normal for age (40–45 by age)		1.3/0.61	
≥ 70	5.8/0.75		
Work of breathing			
Accessory muscle use	2.2/0.42		
Moderate/severe retractions		3.2/0.76	
Chest radiograph			
Atelectasis	10.5/0.81		
Abnormal		1.2/0.73	

Risk factors are presented as positive or negative likelihood ratios (+ LR/– LR). The likelihood ratio can be multiplied by the pre-test odds (ratio of the risk/1-risk) to obtain the post-test odds. For example, with a prior risk of hospitalisation of 33% (odds of 0.33/0.66 = 0.5), a finding with a positive LR of 4 increases the odds to 2, corresponding to a post-test risk of 67% (2/2+1).
*Severe disease defined as unable to maintain alert, active and well-hydrated while taking oral fluids throughout their illness.

investigators, in particular the Canadian multicentre PICNIC study, which included a broad cohort of 689 children hospitalised for respiratory syncytial virus during the 1990s, have attempted to predict severe disease defined as intensive care unit admission, mechanical ventilation, or mortality.[18] A number of large, prospective studies are currently underway, and much more data will be available in the next few years.

Risk for severe disease has consistently been associated with the presence of underlying chronic illness including congenital heart disease, chronic lung disease, prematurity, and immunodeficiency. The risk for morbidity in high-risk infants has declined over recent decades[23] and may be further lowered by new preventive immune therapies such as palivizumab, which has been shown to reduce hospitalisation rates for respiratory syncytial virus in some high-risk sub-groups.[24] The cost–benefit assessment of these therapies is controversial and recommendations for their use vary internationally.[1,2]

Young age (defined variably in studies as less than 6–12 weeks) has also been identified as a risk factor for severe disease. In one study of infants followed after an emergency department visit for bronchiolitis, 55% of those under 3 months of age went on to have severe disease (defined as not alert and active through the illness or unable to maintain hydration on oral fluids) compared with 28% of older infants.[17] A recent, large, multicentre study by Mansbach et al.[22] prospectively enrolled 1456 children under 2 years of age presenting to an emergency department with bronchiolitis. In this study, infants less than 2 months of age were hospitalised at a significantly higher rate compared to older infants (77% versus 36%; $P < 0.001$).[22] Apnoea is a specific concern for young infants although recent research suggests that the incidence may be low and limited to a defined high-risk group. A retrospective study of 691 infants under 6 months of age who were hospitalised for bronchiolitis found that apnoea occurred in 19 (2.7%).[25] All of these apnoeic infants were identified by risk criteria including: (i) a history of an apnoeic episode having already occurred; or (ii) young age defined as age less than one month in full-term infants or, in premature infants, a post-conceptual age less than 48 weeks.

Specific findings on physical examination have been less consistently associated with outcomes of bronchiolitis. Respiratory rate has been predictive in some studies, but not others, and clinical scores have had limited ability to predict disease progression.[17,18] In the Mansbach et al.[22] multicentre study, having only mild or no retractions at initial assessment was associated with a modest, but statistically significant, decrease in the likelihood of being admitted to the hospital (likelihood ratio of 0.76). A likely reason for the limited value of signs and symptoms is the marked variability that is characteristic of bronchiolitis. Transient events such as mucus plugging or nasal obstruction can dramatically affect an infant's respiratory status from moment to moment. Since any diagnostic test must be reliable before it can be predictive, it is not surprising that a single assessment has limited value to predict progression. The variability of bronchiolitis speaks to the importance of re-assessing an infant over a period of time and documenting findings objectively to determine whether there has been a change in clinical status.

OXYGEN AND PULSE OXIMETRY

The appropriate role for pulse oximetry as a tool to assess and predict severity of bronchiolitis has been a topic of controversy. It is clear that mild hypoxaemia (90–95% at sea level) is often not detectable on physical examination but can be measured easily and reliably by pulse oximetry. However, the significance of mild hypoxaemia on short- and long-term outcomes for healthy infants is less certain.[2] Hypoxaemia in bronchiolitis is generally caused by mucus plugging and atelectasis leading to ventilation–perfusion mismatch in the lung. Studies of both in-patients and out-patients have found bronchiolitic infants with hypoxaemia to be more likely to progress to severe disease.[17,18] In the Mansbach *et al.*[22] multicentre study, an initial oxygen saturation of less than 94% increased the likelihood by a factor of 5.4 that the child would eventually be discharged. This threshold was consistent with a survey of American paediatric emergency physicians which found that decreasing the oxygen saturation from 94% to 92% in a clinical vignette correlated with a substantial increase in the likelihood to admit to the hospital.[26]

However, research also suggests that arbitrary thresholds for initiating and maintaining oxygenation may be driving hospital utilisation for bronchiolitis with little evidence of benefit. Reviews of hospitalised infants have found that a substantial proportion of infants remain in the hospital to receive oxygen when other abnormalities have normalised; in one British study, the mean lag for oxygenation to normalise was 66 h after all other problems had resolved.[27] The use of continuous pulse oximetry during observation in the hospital is particularly problematic, as mucus plugging or airway malpositioning may cause transient dips in pulse oximetry readings, which may then lead to re-institution of oxygen in an otherwise improving infant and require a prolonged hospital stay to wean it down. Further evidence is needed in this area, but, basic principles related to the use of pulse oximetry for bronchiolitis were stressed in the 2006 Bronchiolitis Clinical Practice Guideline developed by the American Academy of Pediatrics with input from other specialties and the European Respiratory Society.[2] These principles include:

1. Keeping in mind that physiological changes related to hypoxaemia in healthy infants begin to occur when oxygen saturation falls below 90%.

2. The decision to initiate oxygen should be based on persistent hypoxaemia after checking the placement of the device and initiating simple manoeuvres, such as nasal suctioning and repositioning.

3. When an infant is improving, continuous measurement of pulse oximetry can be discontinued and replaced by spot checks.[2]

THERAPY

Pharmacological therapy for bronchiolitis has been a highly controversial issue with wide variability in practice, in particular for bronchodilators and corticosteroids.[10,11] Since these therapies have proven benefit in asthma, clinicians may extrapolate their efficacy to infants with wheezing, although there are important differences in anatomy and pathophysiology that may lead to a different response. A number of high-quality research studies have recently added to the evidence base for these therapies and are discussed below. In general, current evidence suggests that these and other specific therapies have at best a limited short-term effect in typical cases of bronchiolitis, with no justification for their routine use. Supportive care remains the mainstay of management for infants with bronchiolitis in both the out-patient and in-patient settings, including ensuring adequate hydration and oxygenation and clearance and positioning of the airway.

BRONCHODILATORS

The literature assessing response to bronchodilators among infants with bronchiolitis is extensive and is best approached through systematic reviews such as the regularly updated, high-quality, meta-analyses compiled in the Cochrane Database of Systematic Reviews (see <www.cochrane.org>). These studies can be organised by type of bronchodilator including β_2-agonists (*e.g.* salbutamol/albuterol), combined α/β-agonists (epinephrine), and anticholinergics (ipratropium). The outcomes studied range from short-term response in a clinical score over minutes following administration to clinical outcomes such as admission to the hospital or length of hospitalisation.

The largest number of studies focus on short-term response to β_2-agonists.[28] When changes in clinical scores are pooled across these studies using different protocols and bronchodilators, an overall statistically significant improvement is observed; however, the clinical importance of this change is hard to quantify given the multiple different scores used. Another method of analysis pools together the studies that dichotomised patients into a clinical response versus no response. The graphical representation of this analysis (Fig. 1) illustrates a number of the issues involved in interpreting this body of research. First, there is substantial heterogeneity in the results with positive and negative effects observed. Bronchodilators routinely cause tachycardia and agitation, which can potentially worsen respiratory status in some infants and must be balanced against any potential benefits. Second, many infants (43% overall) in the control groups of these studies showed improvement, likely due to typical variability in clinical status. This is important to recognise in the clinical setting, as an improvement could be attributed to β-agonist effect. Overall, this analysis found a difference in the absolute rate of improvement of 14%, which was statistically significant only in a fixed effects analysis, not the random-effects approach that takes into account variation between studies. Even if this difference is assumed to represent a true effect, it would represent a short-term improvement attributable to the β_2-agonist in only about one out of seven infants treated, with three infants having an improvement unrelated to therapy.

Other bronchodilators have also been assessed for short-term response. Epinephrine is a β_2-agonist with additional α-agonist effects that have been hypothesised to reduce oedema in the airway through vasoconstriction.[29] Multiple studies have compared epinephrine to salbutamol and these have been analysed in a Cochrane review.[29] Overall, four studies in out-patient settings assessed short-term response in clinical score, respiratory rate and other measures and showed a significant improvement with epinephrine treatment compared to salbutamol. In four in-patient studies there was no

Fig. 1 Cochrane Collaboration Systematic Review of studies assessing difference in rate of improvement after β_2-agonist bronchodilators or placebo among children with bronchiolitis. From Gadomski and Bhasale;[28] © Cochrane Collaboration, used with permission.

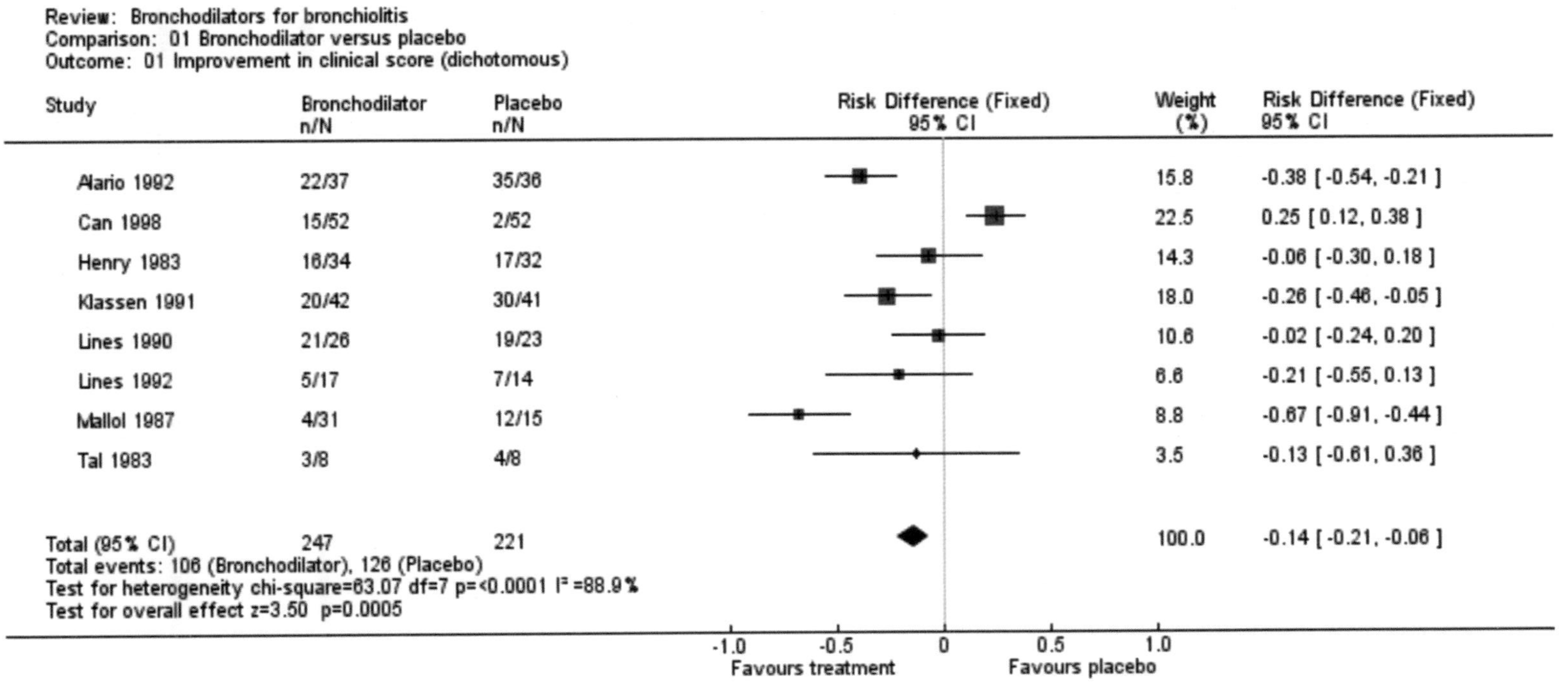

Review: Bronchodilators for bronchiolitis
Comparison: 01 Bronchodilator versus placebo
Outcome: 01 Improvement in clinical score (dichotomous)

Study	Bronchodilator n/N	Placebo n/N	Risk Difference (Fixed) 95 % CI	Weight (%)	Risk Difference (Fixed) 95 % CI
Alario 1992	22/37	35/38		15.8	-0.38 [-0.54, -0.21]
Can 1998	15/52	2/52		22.5	0.25 [0.12, 0.38]
Henry 1983	18/34	17/32		14.3	-0.06 [-0.30, 0.18]
Klassen 1991	20/42	30/41		18.0	-0.26 [-0.46, -0.05]
Lines 1990	21/26	19/23		10.6	-0.02 [-0.24, 0.20]
Lines 1992	5/17	7/14		6.6	-0.21 [-0.55, 0.13]
Mallol 1987	4/31	12/15		8.8	-0.67 [-0.91, -0.44]
Tal 1983	3/8	4/8		3.5	-0.13 [-0.61, 0.36]
Total (95 % CI)	247	221		100.0	-0.14 [-0.21, -0.06]

Total events: 108 (Bronchodilator), 126 (Placebo)
Test for heterogeneity chi-square=63.07 df=7 p=0.0001 I²=88.9 %
Test for overall effect z=3.50 p=0.0005

-1.0 -0.5 0 0.5 1.0
Favours treatment   Favours placebo

difference between therapies in most short-term outcomes. Anti-cholinergic agents such as ipratropium have not been shown to have any efficacy when added to bronchodilators in limited study.

Beyond short-term response in clinical scores, meta-analyses of studies assessing bronchodilator effects on clinical outcomes and duration of illness have almost uniformly found no effect across all settings. Out-patient studies have found no overall reduction in hospitalisation with bronchodilators compared to placebo.[28] The Cochrane meta-analysis of studies comparing salbutamol and epinephrine found no difference in hospitalisation, with a recently conducted trial of 703 children finding only a small benefit favouring albuterol.[30,31] In-patient studies, including a multicentre, randomised trial of epinephrine versus placebo, have found no reduction in duration of hospitalisation.

Overall, the body of evidence on bronchodilators suggests that, if there is a beneficial effect, it is short-term, limited to a subgroup of children, and must be balanced against potential adverse effects. The American Academy of Pediatrics Bronchiolitis Guideline Committee noted the questionable risk–benefit balance of bronchodilators and suggested that they are an option for therapy, but only when a documented response has been observed after treatment so that use is limited to infants who demonstrate benefit.[2]

CORTICOSTEROIDS

Corticosteroids continue to be prescribed regularly for bronchiolitis despite a growing body of evidence suggesting that they are ineffective for a typical infant with a first-time episode of wheezing. A Cochrane meta-analysis of inpatient studies combining over 1100 patients suggests that length of stay in the hospital is not significantly reduced by corticosteroids.[32] One small study of high-dose dexamethasone given in the emergency department had suggested a reduction in hospitalisation rates.[33] However, a recent publication by the US Pediatric Emergency Care Applied Research Network (PECARN) found no difference in admission or clinical score for 600 infants enrolled in a multicentre, randomised, clinical trial.[33,34] The PECARN study also assessed potential subgroups including infants with atopy or family history of asthma and found no benefit of dexamethasone in these children. Most of the studies of corticosteroids in bronchiolitis have focused on previously healthy children with first episode of wheeze and are not generalisable to other clinical scenarios.

OTHER THERAPIES

The role for other therapies in bronchiolitis is limited although small studies suggest a role for future research. Nebulised 3% hypertonic saline has been shown to improve airway clearance in cystic fibrosis, and a recent trial among infants hospitalised with bronchiolitis found a 26% reduction in hospital length of stay compared to a control group who received normal saline.[35] Chest physiotherapy to help clear the airway has not been found to be effective as a routine therapy in limited study.[36]

For infants with severe bronchiolitis, research suggests a potential benefit for continuous positive airway pressure. A recent, randomised trial with a cross-over design found a significant reduction in capillary pCO_2 associated with continuous positive airway pressure when used in a group of 31 infants with bronchiolitis in the intensive care unit.[37] Heliox is another current area of study in the intensive care unit setting and trials have found varying results. Studies focused on clinical scores have found a transient reduction in respiratory distress associated with heliox,[38] although a multicentre, randomised trial of 39 infants found no reduction in the need for positive pressure ventilation compared to oxygen alone.[39] Further study of these therapies is needed.

Antimicrobial agents have a limited role in bronchiolitis. Ribavirin has activity against the respiratory syncytial virus but is not recommended in otherwise healthy infants due to its limited efficacy and high cost; however, it may have a role in immunocompromised children or very severe cases.[2] Antibiotics are often prescribed for infants with bronchiolitis but only have benefit when a documented bacterial co-infection is present. Otitis media is the most common bacterial complication of bronchiolitis, affecting as many as 50–60% of infants at some time in the course of illness, although it can be managed as it would in other clinical situations.[40]

Key points for clinical practice

- Bronchiolitis is a common lower respiratory tract infection affecting a third of children under 2 years of age. Although hospitalisation rates for bronchiolitis have increased, mortality rates remain low.

- Respiratory syncytial virus is the most common cause of bronchiolitis and infects almost all children in the first 2 years of life.

- The clinical course of bronchiolitis includes progression of viral infection from upper to the lower respiratory tract over several days with a prolonged period of recovery lasting weeks in some infants.

- Underlying chronic medical illness (including congenital heart disease, chronic lung disease, prematurity and immunodeficiency) is a risk factor for progression to severe bronchiolitis. These risks may be ameliorated by the development of preventive immunotherapy for respiratory syncytial virus.

- Age less than 2–3 months has been associated with increased risk for severe bronchiolitis, with apnoea as a specific concern for infants under 1 month or premature infants less than 48 weeks' post-conception.

- The predictive value of specific findings on physical examination is limited by the minute-to-minute variability that is characteristic of bronchiolitis and may require a period of observation to obtain an adequate assessment.

- Mild hypoxaemia less than 94% on room air has been associated with an increased rate of progression to severe bronchiolitis although arbitrary cut-off points for maintaining oxygenation may be driving increased hospital utilisation.

(cont'd)

Key points for clinical practice (cont'd)

- When an infant hospitalised with bronchiolitis is improving, continuous pulse oximetry can be discontinued in favour of intermittent measurements.

- Bronchodilators have been associated with transient improvement in a subset of infants with bronchiolitis although they do not impact the overall course of illness. If prescribed, bronchodilators should be limited to infants who demonstrate a beneficial response to therapy.

- Corticosteroids are not effective in typical cases of bronchiolitis and should not be prescribed routinely.

- Ribavirin, although effective against respiratory syncytial virus, should be considered only for high-risk and severe cases of bronchiolitis.

- Antibiotics should only be prescribed for documented bacterial infection as a complication of bronchiolitis.

References

1. Yanney MP, Vyas HG. The treatment of bronchiolitis. *Arch Dis Child* 2008; 93: 793798.
2. Subcommittee on Diagnosis and Management of Bronchiolitis. *Pediatrics* 2006; **118**: 1774–1793.
3. Shay DK, Holman RC, Roosevelt GE, Clarke MJ, Anderson LJ. Bronchiolitis-associated mortality and estimates of respiratory syncytial virus-associated deaths among US children, 1979–1997. *J Infect Dis* 2001; **183**: 16–22.
4. Leader S, Kohlhase K. Recent trends in severe respiratory syncytial virus (RSV) among US infants, 1997 to 2000. *J Pediatr* 2003; **143 (Suppl)**: S127–S132.
5. Mansbach JM, McAdam AJ, Clark S *et al*. Prospective multicenter study of the viral etiology of bronchiolitis in the emergency department. *Acad Emerg Med* 2008; **15**: 111–118.
6. Hall CB. Respiratory syncytial virus and parainfluenza virus. *N Engl J Med* 2001; **344**: 1917–1928.
7. Kotaniemi-Syrjanen A, Vainionpaa R, Reijonen TM, Waris M, Korhonen K, Korppi M. Rhinovirus-induced wheezing in infancy – the first sign of childhood asthma? *J Allergy Clin Immunol* 2003; **111**: 66–71.
8. Kahn JS. Epidemiology of human metapneumovirus. *Clin Microbiol Rev* 2006; **19**: 546–557.
9. Schuh S, Lalani A, Allen U *et al*. Evaluation of the utility of radiography in acute bronchiolitis. *J Pediatr* 2007; **150**: 429–433.
10. Christakis DA, Cowan CA, Garrison MM, Molteni R, Marcuse E, Zerr DM. Variation in inpatient diagnostic testing and management of bronchiolitis. *Pediatrics* 2005; **115**: 878–884.
11. Behrendt CE, Decker MD, Burch DJ, Watson PH. International variation in the management of infants hospitalized with respiratory syncytial virus. International RSV Study Group. *Eur J Pediatr* 1998; **157**: 215–220.
12. Bordley WC, Viswanathan M, King VJ *et al*. Diagnosis and testing in bronchiolitis: a systematic review. *Arch Pediatr Adolesc Med* 2004; **158**: 119–126.
13. Perlstein PH, Kotagal UR, Bolling C *et al*. Evaluation of an evidence-based guideline for bronchiolitis. *Pediatrics* 1999; **104**: 1334–1341.
14. Henrickson KJ, Hall CB. Diagnostic assays for respiratory syncytial virus disease. *Pediatr Infect Dis J* 2007; **26**: S36–S40.
15. Macartney KK, Gorelick MH, Manning ML, Hodinka RL, Bell LM. Nosocomial respiratory syncytial virus infections: the cost-effectiveness and cost-benefit of infection control. *Pediatrics* 2000; **106**: 520–526.
16. Levine DA, Platt SL, Dayan PS *et al*. Risk of serious bacterial infection in young febrile

infants with respiratory syncytial virus infections. *Pediatrics* 2004; **113**: 1728–1734.

17. Shaw KN, Bell LM, Sherman NH. Outpatient assessment of infants with bronchiolitis. *Am J Dis Child* 1991; **145**: 151–155.

18. Wang EE, Law BJ, Stephens D. Pediatric Investigators Collaborative Network on Infections in Canada (PICNIC) prospective study of risk factors and outcomes in patients hospitalized with respiratory syncytial viral lower respiratory tract infection. *J Pediatr* 1995; **126**: 212–219.

19. Swingler GH, Hussey GD, Zwarenstein M. Randomised controlled trial of clinical outcome after chest radiograph in ambulatory acute lower-respiratory infection in children. *Lancet* 1998; **351**: 404–408.

20. Swingler GH, Hussey GD, Zwarenstein M. Duration of illness in ambulatory children diagnosed with bronchiolitis. *Arch Pediatr Adolesc Med* 2000; **154**: 997–1000.

21. Voets S, van Berlaer G, Hachimi-Idrissi S. Clinical predictors of the severity of bronchiolitis. *Eur J Emerg Med* 2006; **13**: 134–138.

22. Mansbach JM, Clark S, Christopher NC et al. Prospective multicenter study of bronchiolitis: predicting safe discharges from the emergency department. *Pediatrics* 2008; **121**: 680–688.

23. Navas L, Wang E, de Carvalho V, Robinson J. Improved outcome of respiratory syncytial virus infection in a high-risk hospitalized population of Canadian children. Pediatric Investigators Collaborative Network on Infections in Canada. *J Pediatr* 1992; **121**: 348–354.

24. Romero JR. Palivizumab prophylaxis of respiratory syncytial virus disease from 1998 to 2002: results from four years of palivizumab usage. *Pediatr Infect Dis J* 2003; **22 (Suppl)**: S46–S54.

25. Willwerth BM, Harper MB, Greenes DS. Identifying hospitalized infants who have bronchiolitis and are at high risk for apnea. *Ann Emerg Med* 2006; **48**: 441–447.

26. Mallory MD, Shay DK, Garrett J, Bordley WC. Bronchiolitis management preferences and the influence of pulse oximetry and respiratory rate on the decision to admit. *Pediatrics* 2003; **111**: e45–e51.

27. Unger S, Cunningham S. Effect of oxygen supplementation on length of stay for infants hospitalized with acute viral bronchiolitis. *Pediatrics* 2008; **121**: 470–475.

28. Gadomski AM, Bhasale AL. Bronchodilators for bronchiolitis. *Cochrane Database Syst Rev* 2006; 3: CD001266.

29. Hartling L, Wiebe N, Russell K, Patel H, Klassen TP. Epinephrine for bronchiolitis. *Cochrane Database Syst Rev* 2004 (1): CD003123.

30. Walsh P, Caldwell J, McQuillan KK, Friese S, Robbins D, Rothenberg SJ. Comparison of nebulized epinephrine to albuterol in bronchiolitis. *Acad Emerg Med* 2008; **15**: 305–313.

31. Hartling L, Wiebe N, Russell K, Patel H, Klassen TP. A meta-analysis of randomized controlled trials evaluating the efficacy of epinephrine for the treatment of acute viral bronchiolitis. *Arch Pediatr Adolesc Med* 2003; **157**: 957–964.

32. Patel H, Platt R, Lozano JM, Wang EE. Glucocorticoids for acute viral bronchiolitis in infants and young children. *Cochrane Database Syst Rev* 2004 (3): CD004878.

33. Schuh S, Coates AL, Binnie R et al. Efficacy of oral dexamethasone in outpatients with acute bronchiolitis. *J Pediatr* 2002; **140**: 27–32.

34. Corneli HM, Zorc JJ, Majahan P et al. A multicenter, randomized, controlled trial of dexamethasone for bronchiolitis. *N Engl J Med* 2007; **357**: 331–339.

35. Kuzik BA, Al-Qadhi SA, Kent S et al. Nebulized hypertonic saline in the treatment of viral bronchiolitis in infants. *J Pediatr* 2007; **151**: 266–270.

36. Webb MS, Martin JA, Cartlidge PH, Ng YK, Wright NA. Chest physiotherapy in acute bronchiolitis. *Arch Dis Child* 1985; **60**: 1078–1079.

37. Thia LP, McKenzie SA, Blyth TP, Minasian CC, Kozlowska WJ, Carr SB. Randomised controlled trial of nasal continuous positive airways pressure (CPAP) in bronchiolitis. *Arch Dis Child* 2008; **93**: 45–47.

38. Cambonie G, Milesi C, Fournier-Favre S et al. Clinical effects of heliox administration for acute bronchiolitis in young infants. *Chest* 2006; **129**: 676–682.

39. Liet JM, Millotte B, Tucci M et al. Noninvasive therapy with helium-oxygen for severe bronchiolitis. *J Pediatr* 2005; **147**: 812–817.

40. Andrade MA, Hoberman A, Glustein J, Paradise JL, Wald ER. Acute otitis media in children with bronchiolitis. *Pediatrics* 1998; **101**: 617–619.

Matthew E. Abrams

3

Hydrops fetalis

A sign is defined within medicine as any objective evidence of disease. Hydrops fetalis is one of the most difficult signs one encounters in neonatal perinatal medicine. The presence of hydrops or excess fluid accumulations always indicates the presence of disease. There is almost no other sign or symptom one deals with in the newborn that is associated with so many different diagnoses. Trying to find the underlying aetiology can be challenging and take months to years with some cases remaining idiopathic.

Hydrops has been reported to complicate as many as 1 in 1700 pregnancies. Although uncommon, these infants are often very ill and make up as much as 3% of perinatal mortality. The earlier in pregnancy that hydrops is diagnosed, the higher the mortality with diagnosis before 20 weeks' gestation carrying mortality rates > 90%.[1]

In its strictest sense, hydrops fetalis is defined as abnormal fluid accumulation in more than one area of the fetus. This may include the amniotic fluid and the placental compartments. It occurs due to some underlying disease process causing an imbalance in the mechanisms which intricately control the flux of fluid in and out of tissues. In addition, most of the literature is based on case reports making it difficult to differentiate association from causality of disease. Depending on what part of the world one is born, immune hydrops due to iso-immunisation with the Rhesus blood group is now relatively uncommon and mostly preventable. Most cases are now due to non-immune causes. Probably the most significant advancement in the last 10–15 years has been the better recognition and ability to diagnosis underlying metabolic disorders in these babies. Evaluating these infants and making a diagnosis must be well planned and systematic.

Matthew E. Abrams MD FAAP
Pediatrix Medical Group, Phoenix Perinatal Associates, Division of Neonatal Medicine, 1919 E. Thomas, Bldg 'C', Phoenix, AZ 85016, USA
E-mail: matthew_abrams@pediatrix.com

Case example

A 33 week and 4 day gestational-age female infant was delivered by caesarean delivery for preterm labour and worsening hydrops fetalis. Antenatally, the fetus was noted on a 28-week ultrasound to have hydrops marked by significant ascites and bilateral pleural effusions. There were no other obvious fetal anomalies. Amniocentesis was performed for chromosomal analysis which was normal. Percutaneous umbilical blood sampling was performed and revealed a haematocrit of 32%. Titres for congenital infections were negative. Prior to delivery, 500 ml of clear yellow fluid was drained from the fetal abdomen to facilitate delivery and reduce immediate respiratory compromise. After birth, the infant had significant respiratory distress requiring intubation and mechanical ventilation. On examination, she was noted to have coarse facies, hypertelorism, hepatomegaly, splenomegaly, and significant ascites. Initial laboratory investigation revealed an elevated direct bilirubin level, and elevated γ-glutamyl transpeptidase level, haematocrit of 35% and reticulocyte count of 8.5%. The initial platelet count was normal and the remainder of the liver function tests was initially normal. The initial abdominal ultrasound revealed significant ascites and hepatomegaly. The head ultrasound and echocardiogram were normal. Because of severe ascites and respiratory difficulty, paracentesis was performed shortly after birth. Pathological examination of the peritoneal fluid and peripheral blood smear revealed vacuolated lymphocytes, which suggested a metabolic disorder.[2] Further evaluation revealed an elevated sialic acid level consistent with the diagnosis of infantile sialic acid storage disease. Chromosomal testing and testing for Noonan syndrome were also negative. Multiple care conferences were held with the family to discuss the poor chance of survival and possible withdrawal of support since the infant had failed extubation multiple times.[3–10] Ultimately, the infant deteriorated and was withdrawn from support at 34 days of life. Cultures from the day prior to death revealed a concurrent Gram-negative urinary tract infection.

The above case illustrates a number of key points in the investigation of infants with hydrops fetalis. Since fluid accumulations were in two unrelated body cavities, the likelihood of the presence of systemic disease was very high. Prenatal testing was able essentially to rule out cardiac disease, major chromosomal anomalies, major anatomical defects, common congenital infections, and severe fetal anaemia as aetiologies for hydrops. In addition, evaluations in the first hours of life, including a detailed physical examination, were able to narrow the possible aetiologies further.

PATHOPHYSIOLOGY

What causes the abnormal fluid accumulation in tissues is dependent on the disruption of normal physiology by the underlying diagnosis. Fluid accumulation in body compartments is dependent on the fluid going in and out of those compartments. In essence, hydrops occurs due to an imbalance of the mechanisms which regulate fluid passage in and out of the tissues. Any disease that disrupts the normal tightly controlled mechanisms can result in abnormal fluid collection in tissues. In addition, many of the diseases may cause hydrops by multiple mechanisms. A thorough discussion of the physiology of the microcirculation and lymphatic system is beyond the scope of this chapter. The reader is referred to *The Textbook of Medical Physiology* by Guyton and Hall and *Diseases of the Lymphatics* by Browse, Burnand, and Mortimer.[11,12] Once one sees the complex physiology that regulates the capillary and lymphatic system, it is evident how difficult the evaluation and diagnosis of infants with hydrops may be.

The microcirculation of the different organs and tissues in the body is organised specifically to serve that organ's needs. Blood flow to and from capillaries and the diffusion between the capillary and interstitial fluid spaces are tightly controlled and are different in each tissue. In addition, blood flow does not flow continuously through the capillaries. The flow is intermittent, occurring every few seconds to minutes through a process called vasomotion.[12]

The interstitium, or spaces between cells, and the fluid in this space, the interstitial fluid, constitutes about one-sixth of the total volume of the body. This area is full of proteoglycan filaments which make it difficult for fluid to flow easily through the interstitium. Since most fluid is normally entrapped within the tissue gel of the interstitium, very little fluid is free flowing. However, when tissue oedema develops, more fluid becomes free flowing.[12]

In summary, the causes of increased fluid accumulation in tissues are:[12,13]

1. *Increased capillary hydrostatic pressure.*

2. *Decreased interstitial fluid hydrostatic pressure which is mainly regulated by the pumping of the lymphatic system.*

3. *Decreased plasma colloid osmotic pressure which is regulated by the proteins, of the plasma and interstitial fluids.*

4. *Increased interstitial fluid colloid osmotic pressure, which is normally much lower than the plasma colloid osmotic pressure.*

5. *Increased capillary permeability.*

6. *Impaired placental clearance of excess fetal fluid.*

THE LYMPHATIC SYSTEM

One can see that there are multiple mechanisms within the lymphatic system that may be disrupted to cause abnormal fluid collections. The lymphatic system is important in regulating the volume of interstitial fluid, the pressure of the interstitial fluid, and the concentration of proteins in the interstitial fluids. Lymphatic vessels drain excess fluid directly from the interstitial spaces into the blood stream. Lymphatic vessels from the lower part of the body, left side of the head, left arm and chest region empty into the thoracic duct which then drains into the venous system at the juncture of the left internal jugular vein and the left subclavian vein. The right side of the head, right arm, and right side of the chest are drained by the right lymphatic duct into the venous system at the junction of the right subclavian vein and the internal jugular vein. Lymphatics have valves at the tips of the lymphatic capillaries as well as valves along their larger vessels. Backflow closes these valves. Fluid that is not moved through these vessels normally, will begin to accumulate and cause a back pressure into the interstitial spaces. Normally, when the lymphatic

Table 1 Partial list of conditions which may cause or have been associated with hydrops in the newborn

CARDIAC ABNORMALITIES

Arrhythmias
- Supraventricular tachycardia
- Congenital heart block
- Atrial flutter
- Severe sinus bradycardia
- Wolff–Parkinson–White syndrome

Congenital heart disease
- Ebstein's anomaly
- Hypoplastic left heart
- Hypoplastic right heart
- Aortic valve atresia or severe stenosis
- Pulmonary valve atresia
- Teratology of Fallot
- Complex congenital heart disease
- Severe co-arctation of the aorta
- Mid-aortic syndrome (severe co-arctation of the intra-abdominal aorta)

Other cardiovascular lesions
- Cardiomyopathy
- Myocarditis
- Pericarditis
- Cardiac tumours: intrapericardial teratoma, rhabdomyoma, haemangioma, myxoma, and rhabdoid

CONGENITAL INFECTIONS
- Cytomegalovirus
- Parvovirus B19
- Toxoplasmosis
- Rubella
- Syphilis
- Chorio-amnionitis with or without intra-uterine bacterial sepsis
- Herpes simplex virus

HAEMATOLOGICAL DISORDERS
- Anaemia
- Erythroblastosis fetalis (due to Rhesus haemolytic disease)
- Spherocytosis type 1
- α- and β-Thalassemia
- Pyruvate kinase deficiency
- Diamond–Blackfan anaemia

METABOLIC DISORDERS
- Lysosomal storage diseases: mucopolysaccharidosis (MPS) VII and
- IVA, type 2 Gaucher disease, sialidosis, GMI gangliosidosis, galactosialidosis, Niemann–Pick disease type C, disseminated
- Lipogranulomatosis (Farber disease), infantile free sialic acid storage disease (ISSD), and mucolipidosis II (I-cell disease)
- Carbohydrate-deficient glycoprotein syndrome type 1a
- Glucose-6-phosphate isomerase deficiency
- Morquio disease type A
- Neuraminidase deficiencies
- Smith–Lemli–Opitz syndrome
- Transaldolase deficiency
- Congenital disorder of glycosylation (CDG)

Table 1 *(continued)* Partial list of conditions which may cause or have been associated with hydrops in the newborn

CHROMOSOMAL ABERRATIONS
•   Turner syndrome (45,X)
•   Trisomy 21
•   Trisomy 18
•   Tetraploidy
•   Tetrasomy 12q
•   Mitochondrial tRNAGLU gene mutation m.14709T>C
OTHER
•   Congenital hypothyroidism
•   Congenital lymphatic dysplasia
TUMOURS (NON-CARDIAC)
•   Cystic hygroma
•   Sacrococcygeal teratoma
•   Mediastinal teratoma
•   Leukaemia
•   Hepatic tumors: haemangioma, mesenchymal haemartoma, hepatoblastoma
•   Neuroblastoma
•   Placental tumours: chorangioma, choriocarcinoma
•   Soft tissue tumours: haemangioma, fibrosarcoma, rhabdoid tumour
•   Renal tumours: congenital mesoblastic nephroma, Wilms' tumour, rhabdoid tumour, clear cell sarcoma
•   Brain tumours: glioblastoma, haemangioma, teratoma
•   Histiocytoses: Langerhans cell histiocytosis, haemophagocytic lymphohistiocytosis
•   Pulmonary tumours: myofibroblastic tumour

vessels are filled and become stretched, the smooth muscles in the wall of the vessels begin to contract and cause a pumping motion. In addition, external compression of the lymphatics by movement such as exercise and contraction of skeletal muscles, can also induce pumping of the lymphatic vessels. Any abnormality in this intricate plumbing system will cause a disruption of the balance of fluid going in and out of tissues.[11,12]

AETIOLOGY

Hydrops is typically classified into immune and non-immune. Table 1 shows an extensive, yet partial, list of diseases that cause or have been associated with hydrops.[13–18] A thorough discussion of all these possible diagnoses is beyond the scope of this chapter. Immune hydrops has historically been caused mainly by Rhesus iso-immunisation but may be caused by other blood group incompatibilities. With advancements in detection and diagnosis and fetal therapy, Rhesus iso-immunisation has become a relatively uncommon cause of hydrops in the newborn.[1,19]

EVALUATION

In some cases of hydrops fetalis, the underlying diagnosis may be identified prior to the onset of hydrops as may occur with congenital heart block, other congenital heart lesions, and masses such as sacrococcygeal teratoma to name a few. Abnormal fluid accumulation in one body cavity such as that which occurs with isolated ascites or isolated hydrothorax should focus on local pathophysiology first and the diagnostic evaluation should be specifically targeted and not include an entire work-up for hydrops. In cases where there is accumulation in more than one body cavity, the investigation should be directed to eliminate the most common and most easy to diagnose diseases.

PRENATAL

1. Complete pregnancy and family history which can aid in the diagnosis of underlying genetic and metabolic diseases.

2. Maternal laboratory evaluation to include: (i) blood type and indirect Coombs antibody screen; (ii) triple screen to evaluate risk of various disorders; and (iii) complete blood count.

3. Complete fetal survey by a physician who specialises in high-resolution fetal ultrasonography.

4. Consultation with a perinatologist to discuss management of the pregnancy and options of termination if diagnosis is made early in pregnancy or if there are significant fetal abnormalities.

5. Consultation with a neonatologist to discuss possible aetiologies as well as indications for delivery, postnatal management, chances of survival and long-term outcomes. Often, the family is surprised about the difficulty in making a diagnosis, potential length of hospital stay and unknown long-term outcomes. Discussion of autopsy should be considered at this time in the event the infant dies.

In addition, the following may be indicated based on the initial evaluation and findings: (i) fetal electrocardiogram and echocardiogram; (ii) fetal chromosome determination by amniocentesis; (iii) evaluation for congenital infection including cytomegalovirus, parvovirus, coxsackie virus, syphilis, herpes simplex virus, and toxoplasmosis, which may include maternal antibody testing and amniotic fluid testing for culture or polymerase chain reaction; (iv) electron microscopy of chorionic villious samples;[20] and (v) metabolic testing of amniotic fluid and fetal blood.[21,22]

POSTNATAL BASICS

1. Complete physical examination of the infant which may be challenging in the case of severe hydrops.

2. Chest radiograph and abdominal radiograph.

3. Complete blood count with peripheral smear and platelet count.

4. Complete metabolic panel with liver and renal function tests.

5. Chromosomal testing as described below.

6. Echocardiogram to assess structure and function, and presence of pericardial fluid.

7 EKG if arrhythmias suspected.

8. Abdominal ultrasound if suspected ascites and to evaluate anatomy. Include renal and pelvic components.

9. Metabolic testing which should include testing for lysosomal storage diseases.

10. In infants in whom lymphatic dysplasia is suspected or in whom a diagnosis has yet to be made, lymphoscintigraphy should be considered.[23]

11. Autopsy if the infant dies. This is not only important for diagnosis of this infant but also for genetic counselling for the family. The importance of autopsy should be discussed early with the parents as this can more difficult for the family to understand and discuss at the time of death.

These infants are best cared for at centres than can provide neonatal intensive care and have access to specialists that may be needed in the evaluation and management. Infants with severe hydrops will likely have severe respiratory distress and may require high-frequency ventilation. Therefore, a neonatologist and neonatal intensive care team should be present at the delivery. These infants may be very difficult to intubate due to rigidity of the mouth and airway due to severe tissue oedema. Infants with severe hydrops are also at risk for pulmonary hypoplasia and decreased lung compliance which increases their risk for pneumothoraces. In addition to standard equipment for neonatal resuscitation, equipment for emergent thoracentesis, chest tube placement, paracentesis, pericardiocentesis, and umbilical line placement should be readily available in the delivery room.

For infants in whom a diagnosis was not made *in utero* or if hydrops was unexpected, the work-up should be well planned and systematic. The most important part of the initial evaluation is a physical examination. Early consultation with a geneticist is also recommended to assist with the delineation of any dysmorphic features and to lead the genetic and metabolic evaluation. The cardiovascular examination should assess for arrhythmia, evidence of cardiac dysfunction, and evidence of congenital heart disease. Examination of the abdomen is important to assess for ascites, hepatomegaly, splenomegaly, and any masses.

An echocardiogram is important to delineate the anatomy as well as cardiac function and to rule out any significant pericardial effusion. An EKG should be obtained if there is any suspicion of an arrhythmia.

Basic laboratory evaluation

This includes a haematocrit/haemoglobin to evaluate for anaemia, platelet count to evaluate for thrombocytopenia, prothrombin time (PT), partial thromboplastin time (PTT), fibrinogen, and D-dimer to assess for disseminated intravascular coagulation and to assess liver function, a complete metabolic panel to assess renal and liver function as well as to assess for any significant electrolyte abnormalities. A white blood cell count and differential with a peripheral smear should be performed as well.

Infection

Any fluid aspirate can be sent for polymerase chain reaction and culture. Urine can be sent for cytomegalovirus culture or rapid cytomegalovirus antigen testing if available. Some clinicians recommend sending a total IgM to assess for evidence of a congenital infection, although the usefulness of this is not clear and it is not specific. Liver function tests and complete blood counts can also aid in the assessing the likelihood of an infection. Acute late-onset fetal hydrops can also occur with intra-uterine bacterial sepsis. Blood for bacterial culture should be sent in these cases.

Genetic

Blood should be sent for chromosomal analysis and consultation with a geneticist is recommended. A rapid karyotype can be performed to assess for any major chromosomal abnormalities such as Trisomy 21, Trisomy 18, Trisomy 13, Turner's syndrome (45,X), or Klinefelter (47, XXY). High-resolution screening may be needed as well because there also exist a number of microdeletion syndromes that will not initially be detected on routine chromosomal screening. There are also submicroscopic deletions which cannot be detected by routine chromosomal analysis. Fluorescence *in situ* hybridisation (FISH) must be performed. In FISH, there is a DNA probe in which a unique segment of DNA is tagged with a fluorescent substance. This probe fails to attach if the suspected area of DNA is missing. The clinician must suspect a specific diagnosis and a probe must exist for that diagnosis.[24]

There also exist a number of genetic diseases caused by uniparental disomy. Uniparental disomy occurs when both pairs of one's chromosomes originate from the same parent. Genomic imprinting results from genes being turned on or off depending on whether the gene is transmitted through the mother or father.[24]

Metabolic

With improvements in recognition and testing, more and more metabolic diseases are being diagnosed in babies with hydrops fetalis. Previously, many infants would go undiagnosed. In those who died, it was a challenge not being able to counsel the family as to why their baby died and future reproductive risks. In addition, in those infants who survived, it was also a challenge to counsel the family regarding the long prognosis in their infant. Table 2 outlines

Table 2 Laboratory studies for an infant suspected of having an inborn error of metabolism[36]

• Complete blood count with differential and peripheral smear
• Urinalysis
• Blood gases
• Serum electrolytes
• Blood glucose
• Plasma ammonia
• Urine reducing substances
• Urine ketones if acidosis or hypoglycaemia present
• Plasma and urine amino acids, quantitative
• Urine organic acids
• Plasma lactate

the investigation of suspected metabolic disease. Increasingly, lysosomal storage diseases are being recognised in infants that would have previously been diagnosed with idiopathic hydrops. At least 10 different lysosomal storage diseases that have been associated with hydrops.[25-35] Lysosomal disorders are among the few causes of non-immune hydrops fetalis in which a recurrence risk can be ascertained. With an early and accurate diagnosis, genetic counselling and family planning can be offered in these difficult cases.[36]

If one of these disorders is suspected, urine screening tests for mucopolysaccharides and oligosaccharides should be performed. Negative results do not rule out the possibility of a storage disorder and false-positive mucopolysaccharide test results can occur in neonates. The definitive diagnosis of most lysosomal storage disorders is made by appropriate biochemical studies on leukocytes or cultured skin fibroblasts.[36]

POST-NATAL MANAGEMENT

Management of hydrops itself is mainly supportive. The acute management mainly deals with stabilising the infant's respiratory status. Intubation may be difficult; therefore, it is recommended that a neonatologist be present at delivery. In addition, one should anticipate the possible need for emergency thoracentesis, paracentesis, and pericardiocentesis.

For infants with significant ascites or pleural effusions, this may involve on-going fluid aspirations to improve pulmonary compliance. However, removal of these compartmental fluid accumulations does not fix the problem and can cause acute fluid shifts, electrolyte imbalances, and protein loss. If an infant has ascites but is not having respiratory embarrassment or feeding intolerance, regardless of the degree of ascites, repeated paracentesis is not recommended. Significant pleural effusions are more likely to require on-going fluid removal because of direct compression on the lungs. Significant pericardial effusions are going to be very problematic and likely lethal. Somatostatin (Octreotide) has been tried with varied success in treating persistent chylothorax and ascites. However, there is very little data regarding its effectiveness and safety in neonates. It seems to be more effective when these occur due to trauma.[37-39]

Since these infants may have in-dwelling catheters, compromised immune systems, and may be exposed to repeated courses of antibiotics, they should be monitored closely for infections. Without documented evidence of infection, prolonged courses of antibiotics should be avoided as this will not improve the infant's condition and only put the baby at further risk for antibiotic-resistant nosocomial infections.

Nutritional management of these babies can also be challenging. Some of these infants require prolonged parenteral nutrition with all of its possible complications. Enteral nutrition is often challenging since many of these infants will have problems with absorption and lymphatic processing. In infants who cannot tolerate breast-milk because of re-accumulation of ascites or chylothorax, defatted breast-milk or low-fat formulas high in medium-chain triglyderides with intravenous intralipid supplementation may be considered. The safety and efficacy of these strategies is also not well established and are always nutritionally suboptimal compared to human milk. Because of the well-established health benefits of breast-milk, it is the author's opinion that a trial of the mother's milk should always be done prior to utilising any other nutritional regimen.

OUTCOMES

Lallemand et al.,[40] in a review of 94 cases of non-immune hydrops, were able to make a diagnosis in two-thirds of the cases and a suspected diagnosis in an additional 23% of the cases. The most common causes of non-immune hydrops were chromosomal abnormalities (33%), infections (16%), and cardiac pathology (13.8%).[40] Another study[41] from the early 1990s showed similar results with 45,X karyotype and autosomal trisomy compromising 30% of the cases. Additionally, 14% were diagnosed with a congenital infection.[41]

Another series studied cases of hydrops fetalis in a cohort of pregnancies referred to a tertiary maternal fetal medicine centre in the UK,[42] where 12.7% of the 63 cases were associated with an immune cause and 87.3% were of non-immune aetiology. The most common non-immune causes were aneuploidies, parvovirus B19, and primary hydrothorax. A diagnosis was not made in 14.5% of the cases.[42]

For cases of hydrops fetalis diagnosed early in pregnancy, the prognosis is grim. Has,[43] in a review of 30 cases diagnosed in the first trimester, reported that all pregnancies with non-immune hydrops resulted in abortion, intra-uterine fetal death, or termination of the pregnancy. Of the reported cases, 83.3% were found to have a structural abnormality of which cystic hygroma was the most common; in addition, 47.3% of the cases had chromosomal abnormalities.[43] In infants who require fetal blood transfusions, survival may be as high as 98% if there is reversal of hydrops. However, survival rates are much lower in infants with severe hydrops and in those in whom hydrops does not resolve.[44] Long term, those babies that survive appear to do very well.[45] Fetuses with pleural effusions and hydrops treated with thoraco-abdominal shunts may have a 57% chance of survival.[46] In fetuses with non-immune ascites, mortality rates vary depending on the underlying aetiology. Those with metabolic causes carry the highest mortality and fetuses with isolated ascites have the best outcome. Infants with urinary ascites had the best outcomes. Mortality is highest the earlier in pregnancy it is diagnosed and if it is associated with hydrops.[47]

Liu et al.[48] performed a retrospective review of 17 live-born cases of hydrops fetalis. Most cases presented with ascites (70.6%) and cardiomegaly (47%) and 41.2% of the neonates had cardiovascular anomalies. The overall mortality rate was 59%. In comparison with survival cases, those that died were diagnosed earlier, had lower Apgar scores, had more severe acidosis, and had pericardial effusion.[48] Simpson et al.[49] studied 30 cases of non-immune hydrops fetalis in a retrospective review. An aetiology was found in 66% of the cases and only 33% survived to discharge. Poor condition at birth was a strong predictor of death.[49]

In 2007, Huang et al.[50] reported on a retrospective review of 28 live-born neonates. Most of the patients had pleural effusions and ascites. Overall survival rate was 50% and was highest among infants with lymphatic defects. The most significant risk factors for death were younger gestational age and lower serum albumin level.[50] Another retrospective review[51] of 41 babies with hydrops fetalis found an overall mortality rate of 49% with a mean survival time of 15 days. The use of antenatal steroids, surfactant, and high-frequency ventilation did not seem to alter survival rates. Only 10% of the patients had a diagnosis of immune hydrops.[51]

Also in 2007, Abrams *et al.*[19] published a retrospective review of 598 live-born neonates admitted to neonatal intensive care units with the diagnosis of hydrops fetalis. The most common associated diagnoses were congenital heart problems (13.7%), abnormalities in heart rate (10.4%), twin-to-twin transfusion syndrome (9%), congenital anomalies (8.7%), chromosomal abnormalities (7.5%), congenital viral infections (6.7%), congenital anaemia (5%), and congenital chylothorax (3.2%). Overall, 26% remained idiopathic at the time of death or discharge. Of interest, none of the neonates was reported to have been diagnosed with a lysosomal storage disorder. This was likely because of failure of recognition and testing and may have accounted for some of the idiopathic cases. Of the 598 neonates that were not transferred to another hospital or to another service, 44.5% died before discharge. Mortality rates were highest among infants with congenital anomalies (57.7%) and lowest among neonates with congenital chylothorax (5.9%). The study sought to identify factors associated with death. Those factors independently associated with death were younger gestational age, low 5-min Apgar score, and need for high levels of support during the first days after birth. The risk of death was highest among those most premature and those most ill after birth.[19] Another recent, but smaller, study showed mortality rates of 40% and 80% of the cases were non-immune.[52]

COUNSELLING OF THE FAMILY

Counselling of the family of an infant with hydrops fetalis is challenging for the healthcare provider. Extensive counselling must be provided to the family prenatally and postnatally to inform them of the difficulties in making a diagnosis and the possibility of a very prolonged hospitalisation. Also, if a genetic cause of hydrops is found, proper counselling regarding risk of recurrence must also be discussed. In addition, the topic of autopsy must be discussed with the family. In infants with multiple anomalies or in whom a diagnosis was not made prior to death, autopsy may be the last opportunity to establish an aetiology for the hydrops. This is important, since some diagnoses have established patterns of inheritance. At the time of a baby's death, the family is unlikely to be focused on future pregnancies or the risk to the rest of their family. Therefore, autopsy discussions are best held prior to the infant's death.

Key points for clinical practice *(see next page)*

Key points for clinical practice

- Hydrops fetalis is a sign of many possible diseases in the newborn.

- Evaluation of a newborn with hydrops fetalis requires a systematic multidisciplinary approach if a diagnosis has not already been made prenatally.

- Despite improvements in neonatal care, overall survival rates do not seem to have significantly improved. This is likely due to the complexity of underlying disorders.

- Delivering a fetus for worsening hydrops may not improve survival since those that are born prematurely appear to do the worst.

- Anticipation of respiratory problems is critical in the initial management and infants with moderate-to-severe hydrops should be ideally delivered at a facility that can provide high-frequency ventilation and inhaled nitric oxide.

- Consultation with a geneticist and metabolic specialist should be initiated early in the neonatal course and, ideally, prenatally.

- Many infants who survive the newborn period may go on to have gastrointestinal and nutritional problems. Some can require months to years of parenteral nutrition and can succumb to its complications.

- These infants are at significant risk of infection due to severity of illness, dysfunction of lymphatic flow and immune regulation, in-dwelling catheters, and central lines.

- Families must counselled that making a diagnosis may be challenging and the chance of survival is greatly dependent on the underlying disorder, severity of the hydrops, gestational age at delivery, and condition at birth. In addition, the infant may be hospitalised for months and diagnostic testing may be extensive with results taking weeks to months to return.

- The difficult, but critical, topic of autopsy must be discussed early in the evaluation.

References

1. Bukowski R, Saade GR. Hydrops foetalis. *Clin Perinatol* 2000; **27**: 1007–1031.
2. Anderson G, Smith VV, Malone M, Sebire NJ. Blood film examination for vacuolated lymphocytes in the diagnosis of metabolic disorders; retrospective experience of more than 2,500 cases from a single centre. *J Clin Pathol* 2005; **58**: 1305–1310.
3. Aula N, Aula P. Prenatal diagnosis of free sialic acid storage disorders (SASD). *Prenat Diagn* 2006; **26**: 655–658.
4. Aula N, Jalanko A, Aula P, Peltonen L. Unraveling the molecular pathogenesis of free sialic acid storage disorders: altered targeting of mutant sialin. *Mol Genet Metab* 2004; **82**: 99–100.
5. Froissart R, Cheillan D, Bouvier R *et al*. Clinical, morphological, and molecular aspects of sialic acid storage disease manifesting in utero. *J Med Genet* 2005; **42**: 829–836.

6. Gopaul KP, Crook MA. The inborn errors of sialic acid metabolism and their laboratory investigation. *Clin Lab* 2006; **52**: 155–169.
7. Parazzini C, Arena S, Marchetti L *et al.* Infantile sialic acid storage disease: serial ultrasound and magnetic resonance imaging features. *Am J Neuroradiol* 2003; **24**: 398–400.
8. Strehle EM. Salla disease and ISSD – what does the future hold? *Mol Genet Metab* 2004; **82**: 99–100.
9. Suwannarat P. Disorders of free sialic acid. *Mol Genet Metab* 2005; **85**: 85–87.
10. Wreden CC, Wlizla M, Reimer RJ. Varied mechanisms underlie the free sialic acid storage disorders. *J Biol Chem* 2005; **280**: 1408–1416.
11. Browse N, Burnand KG, Mortimer PS. *Diseases of the Lymphatics*. London: Hodder Education, 2003.
12. Guyton AC, Hall JE. The microcirculation and the lymphatic system: capillary fluid exchange, interstitial fluid, and lymph flow. In: *Textbook of Medical Physiology,*. 11th edn. Philadelphia, PA: Elsevier Saunders, 2006; chapter 16.
13. Coulter DM. Hydrops fetalis. In: Spitzer AR. (ed) *Intensive care of the fetus and neonate,* 2nd edn. Philadelphia, PA: Mosby, 2005; 149–157.
14. Forouzan I. Hydrops foetalis: recent advances. *Obstet Gynecol* 1997; **52**: 130–138.
15. Hamden AH. Hydrops foetalis. *eMedicine*. Accessed May 2008. Article last updated December 13, 2007.
16. Isaacs H. Fetal hydrops associated with tumors. *Am J Perinatol* 2008; **25**: 43–68.
17. Van Maldergem L, Jauniaux E, Forneau C, Gillerot Y. Genetic causes of hydrops foetalis. *Pediatrics* 1992; **89**: 81–86.
18. Zeltser I, Parness IA, Ko H, Holzman IR, Kamenir SA. Midaortic syndrome in the fetus and premature newborn: a new etiology of nonimmune hydrops foetalis and reversible fetal cardiomyopathy. *Pediatrics* 2003; **111**; 1437–1442.
19. Abrams ME, Meredith KS, Kinnard P, Clark RH. Hydrops foetalis: a retrospective review of cases reported to a large national database and identification of risk factors associated with death. *Pediatrics* 2007; **120**: 84–89.
20. Fowler DJ, Anderson G, Vellodi A, Malone M, Sebire NJ. Electron microscopy of chorionic villus samples for prenatal diagnosis of lysosomal storage disorders. *Ultrastruct Pathol* 2007; **31**: 15–21.
21. Groener JE, de Graaf FL, Poorthuis BJ, Kanhai HH. Prenatal diagnosis of lysosomal storage diseases using fetal blood. *Prenat Diagn* 1999; **19**: 930–933.
22. Piraud M. Froissart R. Mandon G. Bernard A. Maire I. Amniotic fluid for screening of lysosomal storage diseases presenting in utero (mainly as non-immune hydrops fetalis). *Clin Chim Acta* 1996; **248**: 143–155.
23. Bellini C, Boccardo F, Campisi C *et al.* Lymphatic dysplasias in newborns and children: the role of lymphoscintigraphy. *J Pediatr* 2008; **152**: 587–589.
24. Weaver DD. Birth defects and genetic disorders. In: Polin RA, Yoder MC. (eds) *Workbook in Practical Neonatology*, 4th edn. Philadelphia, PA: Saunders Elsevier, 2007; 397–448.
25. Bonduelle M, Lissens W, Goossens A *et al.* Lysosomal storage diseases presenting as transient or persistent hydrops fetalis. *Genet Counsel* 1991: **2**: 227–232.
26. Burin MG, Scholz AP, Gus R *et al.* Investigation of lysosomal storage diseases in non-immune hydrops fetalis. *Prenat Diagn* 2004; **24**: 653–657.
27. Janssens PM, de Groot AN, de Jong JG, Liebrand-van Sambeek ML, Smits A, Wevers RA. Hydrops foetalis as an indication for a systematic investigation into the presence of lysosomal storage diseases [In Dutch with English abstract]. *Ned Tijdschr Geneeskd* 2004; **148**: 264–268.
28. Kattner E, Schafer A, Harzer K. Hydrops fetalis: manifestation in lysosomal storage diseases including Farber disease. *Eur J Pediatr* 1997: **156**: 292–295.
29. Kooper AJ, Janssens PM, de Groot AN *et al.* Lysosomal storage diseases in non-immune hydrops foetalis pregnancies. *Clin Chim Acta* 2006; **371**: 176–182.
30. Lake BD, Young EP, Winchester BG. Prenatal diagnosis of lysosomal storage diseases. *Brain Pathol* 1998; **8**: 133–149.
31. McKenzie FA, Fietz M, Fletcher J, Smith RL, Wright IM, Jaeken J. A previously undescribed form of congenital disorder of glycosylation with variable presentation in siblings: early fetal loss with hydrops fetalis, and infant death with hypoproteinemia. *Am J Med Genet* 2007; **143**: 2029–2034.

32. Molyneux AJ, Blai E, Coleman N. Daish P. Mucopolysaccharidosis type VII associated with hydrops foetalis: histopathological and ultrastructural features with genetic implications. *J Clin Pathol* 1997; **50**: 252–254.
33. Stone DL, Sidransky E. Hydrops foetalis: lysosomal storage disorders *in extremis*. *Adv Pediatr* 1999; **46**: 409–440.
34. Valayannopoulos V, Verhoeven NM, Metion K *et al*. Transaldolase deficiency: a new cause of hydrops foetalis and neonatal multi-organ disease. *J Pediatr* 2006; **149**: 713–717.
35. Venkat-Raman N, Sebire NJ, Murphy KW. Recurrent fetal hydrops due to mucopolysaccharidosis type VII. *Fetal Diagn Ther* 2006; **21**: 250–254.
36. Burton BK. Inborn errors of metabolism in infancy: a guide to diagnosis. *Pediatrics* 1998; **102**; e69-.
37. Bhatia C, Pratap U, Slavik Z. Octreotide therapy: a new horizon in treatment of iatrogenic chyloperitoneum. *Arch Dis Child* 2001; **85**: 234–235.
38. Coulter DM. Successful treatment with Octreotide of spontaneous chylothorax in a premature infant. *J Perinatol* 2004; **24**: 194–195.
39. Huang Q, Jiang ZW, Jiang J, Li N, Li JS. Chylous ascites: treated with total parenteral nutrition and somatostatin. *World J Gastroenterol* 2004; **10**: 2588–2591.
40. Lallemand AV, Doco-Fenzy M, Gaillard DA. Investigation of nonimmune hydrops foetalis: multidisciplinary studies are necessary for diagnosis – review of 94 cases. *Pediatr Dev Pathol* 1999; **2**: 432–439.
41. Boyd PA, Keeling JW. Fetal hydrops. *J Med Genet* 1992; **29**: 91–97.
42. Ismail KM, Martin WL, Ghosh S, Whittle MJ, Kilby MD. Etiology and outcome of hydrops foetalis. *J Matern Fetal Med* 2001; **10**: 175–181.
43. Has R. Non-immune hydrops foetalis in the first trimester: a review of 30 cases. *Clin Exp Obstet Gynecol* 2001; **28**: 187–190.
44. Van Kamp IL, Klumer FJ, Bakkum RS *et al*. The severity of immune fetal hydrops is predictive of fetal outcome after intrauterine treatment. *Am J Obstet Gynecol* 2001; **185**: 668–673.
45. Harper DC, Swingle HM, Weiner CP, Bonthius DJ, Aylward GP, Wildness JA. Long-term neurodevelopmental outcome and brain volume after treatment for hydrops foetalis by *in utero* intravascular transfusion. *Am J Obstet Gynecol* 2006; **195**: 192–200.
46. Picone O, Benachi A, Mandelbrot L, Ruano R, Dumez Y, Dommergues M. Thoracoamniotic shunting for fetal pleural effusions with hydrops. *Am J Obstet Gynecol* 2004; **191**: 2047–2050.
47. Favre R, Dreux S, Dommergues M *et al*. Nonimmune fetal ascites: a series of 79 cases. *Am J Obstet Gynecol* 2004; **190**: 407–412.
48. Liu CA, Huang HC, Chou YY. Retrospective analysis of 17 liveborn neonates with hydrops foetalis [In Chinese with English abstract]. *Chang Gung Med J* 2002; **25**: 826–831.
49. Simpson JH, McDevitt H, Young D, Cameron AD. Severity of non-immune hydrops foetalis at birth continues to predict survival despite advances in perinatal care. *Fetal Diagn Ther* 2006; **21**: 380–382.
50. Huang HR, Tsay PK, Chiang MC, Lien R, Chou YH. Prognostic factors and clinical features in liveborn neonates with hydrops fetalis. *Am J Perinatol* 2007; **24**: 33–38.
51. Wy CAW, Sajous CH, Loberiza F, Weiss MG. Outcome of infants with a diagnosis of hydrops foetalis in the 1990s. *Am J Perinatol* 1999; **16**: 561–567.
52. Trainor B, Tubman R. The emerging pattern of hydrops fetalis – incidence, etiology and management. *Ulster Med J* 2006; **75**: 185–186.

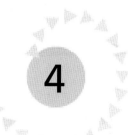

Guy Mitchell

4

Toxic parenting: how parents and other carers can harm children without laying a hand on them

The distinction between public and private law cases is an interesting one. In public law cases (principally Care Proceedings) the family justice system assumes a possible conflict of interests between parent and child and the Court always makes the child a party to the proceedings. The children's guardian looks after the interests of the child, and has responsibility for: (i) the appointment and instruction of a solicitor for the child; (ii) an independent investigation into all the circumstances surrounding the application; and (iii) the preparation of at least one confidential report for the Court with recommendations as to how the child's welfare might best be safeguarded and promoted. In private law cases (mainly arguments between parents about residence and contact) the system assumes no such conflict, the child is not usually made a party to the proceedings, and the role of the children and family reporter is generally less investigative and more facilitative – the task is to get the parents to agree to a child-centred solution. In brief, the focus of public law is the protection of children, and the focus of private law is the promotion of agreement about them.

In many cases, however, there is a great deal of overlap between public and private law cases. It is relatively rare (although by no means unheard of) for physical and sexual abuse to figure in private law cases, and the grosser (and more life-threatening) forms of neglect are hardly the bread and butter of private law contests. But emotional abuse is (in my experience) a very significant factor in many private law disputes. If it is not explicitly alleged by one or other of the parents, it is increasingly recognised by the family justice system as a central feature of at least the more intractable cases. Which is why, in recent years, English courts have increasingly taken to making the child a party even in private law proceedings, and appointing a children's guardian.

Guy Mitchell BA MPhil MSc CQSW
Family Court Adviser, Child and Family Court Advisory and Support Service (CAFCASS), Liverpool, UK
E-mail: guymit@globalnet.co.uk

Most parents in private law proceedings would be horrified to be accused of child abuse. Indeed, I must make it clear that most private law disputes are resolved reasonably quickly and with a fair amount of good will on the part of both parents, who (deep down) are still able to put the child's interests before their own. However, some parents are quite unable to do this, and they will subject the child to years of bitter litigation. For the most part, such parents are oblivious to the severe emotional harm such litigation can cause. If the question is raised, they will often acknowledge the harm and blame the other parent! They will also pretend to themselves that they have only the child's interests at heart.

I believe that the recent blurring of the boundaries between public and private law cases has had much to do with the state's developing awareness of the importance of a child's emotional life. Three systems in particular (the child health system, the child welfare system, and the family justice system) appear finally to have realised what would have been obvious to our grandparents – children's emotional well-being is as important as their physical well-being, unless there is no difference between living and merely existing.

In this chapter, I would like to do five things: (i) to set out, and perhaps improve upon, the definitions of emotional abuse and neglect provided by the Department for Children, Schools and Families (DCSF); (ii) to review the ways in which these forms of harm are expressed at different ages; (iii) to consider the circumstances in which children are most at risk of emotional abuse and neglect; (iv) to review the long-term consequences of emotional abuse and neglect in the absence of timely and effective intervention; and (v) to speculate as to what prevents professionals and the organisations in which they work from providing that timely and effective intervention. I doubt that there will be much here to startle the seasoned practitioner. In a way, that is the point. Emotional abuse and neglect, or toxic parenting, is so common that the danger for professionals is that we are desensitised to it, a theme to which I shall return in due course.

DIFFERENT TITLES

Emotional abuse and neglect has been called many different things. Twenty years ago, we would have been talking about 'maternal deprivation'. It is sometimes referred to as 'emotional ill-treatment' or 'emotional harm'. Alice Miller has called it 'narcissistic disturbance'.[1] Garbarino et al.[2] prefer the title 'psychological maltreatment', arguing that the form of harm we are examining is often unintentional (hence maltreatment rather than ill-treatment), and that it affects all aspects of the way in which a child functions – the way he or she thinks, feels, and chooses. Current UK guidance, as expressed in the third edition of Working Together, distinguishes two forms of harm – 'emotional abuse' and 'neglect'. The distinction is useful but, in practice, the two forms of harm often co-present, which is why, in this chapter, I shall refer to emotional abuse and neglect unless I specifically want to focus upon emotional abuse or neglect.

Emotional abuse

It was a while before the state was willing to acknowledge emotional abuse as a distinct form of harm – and it is not hard to see why. It has proved difficult to operationalise the concept in a way that might command an effective consensus in a pluralistic liberal democracy that tolerates (even if it does not celebrate) a wide range of views as to what constitutes reasonable child care. Emotional abuse in one form or another is so wide-spread that even to name it is to risk opening a Pandora's box. It was not until 1988 that the then Department of Health conceded that emotional abuse might be a distinct form of harm that merited, in certain cases, registration in the same way as physical abuse, sexual abuse and neglect.

The current DCSF defines emotional abuse as:

> *The persistent emotional maltreatment of a child such as to cause severe and persistent adverse effects on the child's emotional development. It may involve conveying to children that they are worthless or unloved, inadequate, or valued only insofar as they meet the needs of another person. It may feature age or developmentally inappropriate expectations being imposed on children. These may include interactions that are beyond the child's developmental capability, as well as overprotection and limitation of exploration and learning, or preventing the child participating in normal social interaction. It may involve seeing or hearing the ill-treatment of another. It may involve serious bullying causing children frequently to feel frightened or in danger, or the exploitation or corruption of children. Some level of emotional abuse is involved in all types of maltreatment of a child, though it may occur alone.*

Neglect

The DCSF defines neglect as:

> *The persistent failure to meet a child's basic physical and/or psychological needs, likely to result in the serious impairment of the child's health or development. Neglect may occur during pregnancy as a result of maternal substance abuse. Once a child is born, neglect may involve a parent or carer failing to provide adequate food and clothing, shelter including exclusion from home or abandonment, failing to protect a child from physical and emotional harm or danger, failure to ensure adequate supervision including the use of inadequate care-takers, or the failure to ensure access to appropriate medical care or treatment. It may also include neglect of, or unresponsiveness to, a child's basic emotional needs.*

This last sentence is an implicit acknowledgement that neglect and emotional abuse are to one another as negative to positive, an observation common to all intelligent attempts to grapple with this difficult subject.

STEPHEN WOLKIND

Stephen Wolkind, focusing exclusively upon emotional abuse, approaches the subject rather differently. He writes:[3]

> I look for three things. First, parental behaviour that is deviant. I use the word 'deviant' in a deliberate form not in any way implying morally wrong but extremely unusual and which from research literature I know to have an adverse effect on a child. Second, I look for a form of child behaviour that is persistently and severely impairing that child's full attainment of mental health. For the child psychiatrist that must be the central factor; the presence of a form of abnormal behaviour which is clearly handicapping. Third, appropriate treatment must have been offered but rejected by the parents.

I have some reservations about all three elements of this definition. As to the first, there is the obvious point that it is not only parents who are guilty of emotional abuse and neglect. Nor do I entirely understand why it is necessary to dodge the question of ethics in the way that Dr Wolkind does here. As to the second point, I have two major reservations about the priority afforded by Dr Wolkind to abnormal behaviour. First, to wait for a child to express such 'abnormal behaviour' whilst observing patently abnormal carer behaviour seems to me to be a counsel of despair. It is not hard to predict, for example, that a baby living with adults whose life-style is characterised by continual drunkenness and violence stands a very good chance of developing 'clearly handicapping' behaviour in due course. Should we not talk of emotional abuse, neglect, or toxic parenting in such circumstances? Second, 'abnormal behaviour' is not necessarily an indication of toxic parenting. Sometimes there is smoke without fire, as every parent out on a bus with an autistic child will need you to know. There is a less than illustrious tradition of automatic inference from difficult child to toxic parent. Witness Bruno Bettelheim's theory of autism[4] and R.D. Laing's theory of schizophrenia.[5]

Even the last part of Dr Wolkind's definition needs some attention. He is surely right to oblige us to work with parents and carers before thinking about (for example) removal. But it is not just the parent or carer who rejects help that is the problem. There is also the parent or carer who is unable (for whatever reason) to benefit from help and advice. Such carers may never actively reject help. But still the children suffer because the carers just can not 'cut it'.

KIERAN O'HAGAN

Kieran O'Hagan, much of whose work should, in my view, be compulsory reading for those involved in working with children and families, distinguishes between emotional and psychological abuse. He defines emotional abuse as 'the sustained, repetitive, inappropriate emotional response to the child's expression of emotion and its accompanying expressive behaviour'. And psychological abuse as 'sustained, repetitive, inappropriate behaviour which damages, or substantially reduces, the creative and developmental potential of crucially important mental faculties and mental processes of a child; these include intelligence, memory, recognition, perception, attention, language and moral development'. I confess that this distinction, of which O'Hagan makes so much in his book,[6] does nothing for me. It may make some kind of intellectual sense but, in practice, it appears to be a distinction without a difference. When you seriously hurt a child's feelings over a long period you affect their feelings, their thinking, and their choices. Similarly, when you damage a child's mental faculties. In reality, these faculties are all connected.

DOROTA IWANIEC

Dorota Iwaniec has written what I consider to be the best book available on the subject of emotional abuse and neglect,[7] which she defines in the following terms:

> Emotional abuse and neglect refer to hostile or indifferent [or misguided] parental behaviour which damages a child's self-esteem, degrades a sense of achievement, diminishes a sense of belonging, and stands in the way of healthy, vigorous and happy development. Emotional abuse is described as overtly rejecting behaviour of carers on the one hand, or as passive neglect on the other.

The parenthesis here is my own interpolation into an otherwise impeccable definition, and I suggest this amendment because I believe that many carers who emotionally abuse or neglect the children for whom they are responsible are neither hostile nor indifferent but very much at sea.

GARBARINO, GUTTMANN AND SEELEY

These workers regard what they call psychological maltreatment as the core of child maltreatment in general, which they define as 'acts of omission or commission by a parent or guardian that are judged by a mixture of community values and professional expertise to be in appropriate and damaging'.[8] This general definition is interesting on two counts. First, it acknowledges that maltreatment is not purely a matter of science. It has to do with expertise, yes. But it also has to do with community values, which are, of course, a site of conflict. Second, it does not depend upon demonstrable harm. True, they do claim that 'in almost all cases, it is the psychological consequences of an act that define that act as abusive'.[9] But later on, they make it clear that 'harmful actions include behaviors that are developmentally dangerous, regardless of whether they have produced visible and measurable harm to the child'.[10] According to these workers, then, the harm to the child does not have to be actual – it can simply be predictable.

Their definition of psychological maltreatment runs as follows:[11]

> Psychological maltreatment is a concerted attack by an adult on a child's development of self and social competence, a pattern of psychically destructive behaviour, and it takes five forms:
>
> • **Rejecting**: (the adult refuses to acknowledge the child's worth and the legitimacy of the child's needs).

- *Isolating*: *(the adult cuts the child off from normal social experiences, prevents the child from forming friendships, and makes the child believe that he or she is alone in the world).*

- *Terrorising*: *(the adult verbally assaults the child, creates a climate of fear, bullies and frightens the child, makes the child believe that the world is capricious and hostile).*

- *Ignoring*: *(the adult deprives the child of essential stimulation and responsiveness, stifling emotional growth and intellectual development).*

- *Corrupting*: *(the adult 'mis-socialises' the child, stimulates the child to engage in destructive antisocial behaviour, reinforces that deviance, and makes the child unfit for normal social relationships.*

These are basic threats to human development.

What attracts me about this definition is the way in which it seeks to break the larger concept of psychological maltreatment down into rather more visible dimensions. The difficulty with more general definitions is that they are usually too broad to operationalise in ways that will command anything like a consensus. But a dimensional definition (I suggest) makes it easier for us all to see what is under our noses and to agree about its significance – at least in the more extreme cases that are likely to come the way of the family justice system.

DANYER GLASER

Dr Danyer Glaser, whose work on sexual abuse and on domestic violence has been widely and deservedly praised, has proposed the following dimensional approach to what I call emotional abuse and neglect and she refers to as 'harmful interactions':[12]

1. *Emotional unavailability, unresponsiveness, and neglect.*
   - *Includes parental insensitivity.*

2. *Negative attributions and misattributions to the child.*
   - *Hostility towards, denigration and rejection of a child who is perceived as deserving these.*

3. *Developmentally inappropriate or inconsistent interactions with the child.*
   - *Expectations of the child beyond her or his developmental capabilities.*
   - *Overprotection and limitation of exploration and learning.*
   - *Exposure to confusing or traumatic events and interactions.*

4. *Failure to recognise or acknowledge the child's individuality and psychological boundary.*
   - *Using the child for the fulfilment of the parent's psychological needs.*
   - *Inability to distinguish between the child's reality and the adults' beliefs and wishes.*

5. *Failing to promote the child's social adaptation.*
   - *Promoting mis-socialisation (including corrupting).*
   - *Psychological neglect (failure to provide adequate cognitive stimulation and/or Author's opportunities for experiential learning.*

AUTHOR'S ATTEMPT TO DEFINE EMOTIONAL ABUSE

All forms of child abuse amount to a kind of emotional abuse, but all the categories put together do not exhaust the possibilities of emotional abuse, and the absence of physical evidence of hurt should not blind us to the existence of the psychological dimension. In very young children, emotional abuse may be obviously expressed in physical ways; in practice, in such cases, the distinction between neglect and emotional abuse may be unhelpful, even unnecessary. With older children, recognition will depend less upon physical symptoms and more upon: (i) close observations of the behaviours of parents and carers; (ii) direct and indirect communications from the child; and (iii) collateral inquiry. As to the second of these, the entire range of behavioural disorders in children may indicate emotional abuse – abnormal aggression, abnormal withdrawal, indiscriminate affection, sleeplessness, night terrors, gorging, food refusal, endless attention-seeking, school problems, sexual dysfunction, and so forth. Perhaps the best way to identify the phenomenon is to consider carefully the behaviour of the parent or carer, if for no other reason than that emotional abuse cannot be automatically inferred from a child's behaviour, how-so-ever disordered that behaviour may appear to be.[13] Quite clearly, then, recognition will be less a medical than a psychosocial procedure. This has implications, not just for the choice of professional, but also for the pace at which that professional must work. I suggest that there are six dimensions to emotional abuse.

Persistent hostility

Some carers hate children. They may hate all children, or just this child. That they hate the child does not necessarily mean that they will be glad to be rid of the child. That hatred may fulfil an important function for the carers in particular, or for the family or school or children's home in particular. As to the former, the child may in some sense be a disappointment – perhaps he or she was not wanted, has a disability, was the 'wrong' sex, or is some kind of reminder of a troubled relationship. As to the latter, most professionals in the people business are familiar with the concept of 'scapegoating', the process whereby one or more members of the group is identified as 'wicked', 'sick', or 'deviant'. That person carries the burden of what else is wrong for, or within, the group, siphoning off aggression that might otherwise be experienced as fatal to the group. She or he becomes the safe place for dumping hatred, the line of least resistance for the malevolent energies with which the system is charged. Often, if the identified patient is removed or expelled from the group, somebody else has to occupy the vacancy.[14] Offers of help from outside may be particularly unwelcome to the persistently hostile carer, precisely because of the vital function performed by the child in question. This form of emotional abuse resembles Garbarino's terrorising and Glaser's negative attributions.

Persistent failure to respond to the child's physical, emotional, intellectual and social needs

Failure to respond to the physical, emotional, intellectual and social needs of a child may take three forms. First, it may be a passive version of persistent hostility. The child may not have to bear the brunt of the carer's terror, but may be all too conscious of getting different treatment from her or his siblings or peers, losing out on treats, affection and encouragement, and being saddled with an unfair burden of household tasks – remember Maria Colwell having to carry home bags of coal which were heavier than she was herself. Second, persistent failure may be the simple consequence of poor parenting skills – remember Jasmine Beckford, whose mother did not know that you have to talk to a child in order for that child to learn to talk! Third, it may be that the carer is incapacitated by illness or disability (physical or mental), or by some form of debilitating addiction. Persistent failure to respond may be intentional or unintentional, conscious or unwitting. This form of emotional abuse resembles Garbarino's rejecting and ignoring and Glaser's emotional unavailability.

Seriously unrealistic expectations

This may be expressed in two ways. First, over-expectation. The carer may expect the baby to sleep all night, to use the potty from birth, never to cry, to go straight to the nipple every time. The carer may: (i) attribute to a very young child intentional malice, cunning and/or defiance; (ii) make quite unreasonable demands upon the child's competence, punishing them for spills, falls, and other accidents; or (iii) make impossible emotional demands of the child, craving parenting instead of offering it. A child may be particularly at risk if she or he lives in a family or institution in which the caring style is characterised by low warmth and high criticism.[15] Second, under-expectation. The carer may resist the child's growing independence, may demand that a young person remain a child for ever, may be overprotective to a degree, and may be jealous of the child's relationships with other children and adults. Under-expecting resembles Garbarino's isolating. I do not think Garbarino's framework offers an adequate understanding of over-expectation. This dimension coincides fairly precisely with Glaser's developmentally inappropriate interactions.

Grossly inappropriate stimulation of a child's aggression or and/or sexuality

A child does not have to be assaulted to suffer from violence.[16] Nor does a child have to be molested to suffer from sexual abuse. A household of violence or hypersexuality may be just as damaging in the long run as are the most direct forms of abuse. This form of emotional abuse has something in common with Garbarino's corrupting. Glaser makes mention of corrupting in connection with her general category of failing to promote the child's social adaptation, but I think that this particular form of emotional abuse merits its own category.

Serious exploitation of a child for the gratification of another's needs

Sexual abuse is an obvious example of this (and other) forms of abuse; however, it is by no means the only one. There is the carer who drives a child to achieve (at whatever the cost) what she or he would like to have achieved. There are the parents who battle with each other through the child, a common enough experience in the breakdown of a marriage or partnership, but frequent, too, when the parents or carers are living together. There are those carers who express their criminality indirectly, through the child, allowing (even forcing) the child to take risks they would not dream of taking themselves – the Fagin phenomenon. The last of these examples recalls Garbarino's corrupting. For the rest, I do not think that Garbarino's framework accounts for this form of emotional abuse. However, this category does have a great deal in common with Glaser's fourth category – failure to recognise or acknowledge the child's individuality and psychological boundary. Under this heading, I should like to highlight two extreme examples which occur from time to time in the family justice system – fabricated or induced illness and parental alienation. The first of these is, thankfully, rare, but when it does occur it is very frightening indeed and requires careful multidisciplinary and interagency assessment and detection.[17] The second, which was described at length by the late Dr Richard Gardner,[18] is quite common in private law contests. There is some controversy as to whether this does or does not involve a mental illness, and even more controversy as to the remedies proposed by Gardner, but the existence of the phenomena that he describes can hardly be doubted. In fabricated illness and parental alienation, we are at the heavy end of toxic parenting.

Grossly inconsistent care

Here, I am thinking of the child who is indulged and abused by turns, who simply does not know whether she or he is loved or loathed. The child who is unable to work out how she or he will be received from one moment to another. The child whose life contains no rhythms, no routines, no stability, no predictability. Such children can take nothing for granted, they can learn no stable boundaries, they may have no sense of their own worth, and no idea as to what is permissible and what forbidden. And their attachments are likely to be at least insecure and, sometimes, downright disorganised. Garbarino's terrorising conveys half of this form of emotional abuse, but does not, I feel, do justice to the essential instability conveyed by the notion of gross inconsistency. Again, this category has something in common with Glaser's developmentally inappropriate or inconsistent interactions, and her idea about the carer's failure to recognise or acknowledge the child's individuality and psychological boundary. However, I would want to emphasise the element of inconsistency here. I suspect that this form of emotional abuse or toxic parenting is amongst the most damaging of all, more damaging even than persistent hostility. I would draw parallels here with three increasingly well-understood phenomena – domestic violence, brain-washing, and the so-called Stockholm syndrome. Common to all three of these extreme situations is the growing and destructive dependence of the victim upon the perpetrator, a defence which Anna Freud first described as identification with the aggressor.[19] Children who have experienced grossly inconsistent care are very difficult to help, partly because the sheer strength of the neurotic bond between them and the carer concerned. These really are the ties that bind a child.

THE EXPRESSION OF EMOTIONAL ABUSE AND NEGLECT

This section reviews some of the ways in which emotional abuse and neglect is expressed during critical stages of childhood – pregnancy, infancy, the pre-school years, primary and secondary school. The *Children Act, 1989* distinction between physical, intellectual, emotional, social and behavioural development is used to structure the observations.[20] Many of the expressions of emotional abuse and neglect are common to all ages, so attention is focused on those that are critical, if not unique, to a particular stage of development.

PREGNANCY

In recent years, much has been learned about the *in utero* development of the fetus in general and of the brain and nervous system in particular. For some time, it has been recognised that the unborn infant is at risk if the mother drinks, takes drugs, or smokes heavily, and it has been strongly suspected that the infant is also at risk if the mother experiences great stress, trauma, or severe depression. Over the last decade or so, these convictions have been thoroughly supported by the science. We can be confident (if that is the right word) that the vicissitudes of intra-uterine existence can have long-term adverse consequences for the child.[21] As Arthur Janov stated:[22] 'It is, therefore, possible to be marked for life even before we see our parents for the first time'. This, of course, is just one of many reasons why we should take seriously the problem of domestic violence. It is also, incidentally, a moment when the phrase 'toxic parenting' ceases to be a metaphor and becomes an all too literal description of what is actually happening to the child.

INFANCY

Emotional abuse and neglect can profoundly harm children of all ages, but the damage done in infancy can be literally life-threatening. As far as physical development is concerned, everyone will be familiar with the infant: (i) who fails to gain weight, length and head circumference at anything like an acceptable rate; (ii) with the pinched, pale and anxious face, the thin and matted hair, the skin that may be dirty and dry in some places, raw and scalding around the groin and bottom; and (iii) who does not meet milestones for sitting, crawling, and babbling. Such children may be left for hours in a push-chair, in a cot, on a sofa, prop-fed from filthy sugar-filled bottles, baby-minded by the television. They may be frequent visitors to accident and emergency departments with recurrent infections of the chest and/or tummy. On the other hand, these are children whose carers are seldom at home to the health visitor and who may be poor attenders at clinic, so that immunisation happens only by dint of determined health visiting.

This is the stage in child development when it is hardest to draw sharp distinctions between physical, intellectual, emotional, social and behavioural aspects. It is also the stage during which the neglect of the physical can have devastating effects upon, in particular, the intellectual and the emotional. The phrase 'toxic parenting' is still depressingly literal: consider just two things – brain development and the development of attachments. The human brain develops in a genetically determined sequence that begins in embryo and is at its most vigorous during the first year of life, although much is still happening up until the age of 4 years. The average human brain weighs 440 g at birth and 1000 g at 4 years of age. During the first 2 years there is serial over-production of axons and dendrites,[23] and there is a corresponding process of myelination.

Blood vessels and support cells (glia) are also developing at a tremendous rate. In the beginning, the connections between the 100 billion cells of the brain (the synapses) are more or less random. They become organised in the context of experience. Each cell can make around 15,000 synaptic connections, and cells can wire up at the rate of 1.8 million connections per second. Where there is severely toxic parenting, either the learning does not happen (if the synapses don't fire they don't wire') or it happens in ways that can have specific and enduring effects upon the brain and potentially devastating effects upon the developing personality.[24] Neuroscience also indicates the literally toxic effects of steroid hormones (such as cortisol) when the infant is exposed to severe and chronic stress.[25] Severe emotional abuse and neglect causes brain damage; however, unlike a blow to the head, this kind of damage is invisible. In order to see it, you have to pay close attention over a period of time; unfortunately, this is precisely what does not happen in so many cases.

It is also known that the first year of life is a crucial period for the development of secure bonds of attachment. Severe emotional abuse and neglect can more or less obliterate the capacity to form secure attachments – it takes no special knowledge or training to work out why. The development of a secure attachment takes the form of a benign song and dance between infant and carer, in which both call and respond to each other, lead and follow each other, in ways that are mutually fulfilling. If the carer fails to call, respond, lead, or follow (or, indeed if the carer does call, respond, lead and follow, but in perverse, hostile, indifferent or unpredictable ways), the chances of the child developing a secure attachment are vanishingly small. In the first year of life, the child can be can brain damaged and its personality wrecked without the carer lifting a finger, always assuming that the process did not start before the child was born.

PRE-SCHOOL YEARS

If a child has experienced severe emotional abuse and neglect throughout infancy, the toddler and pre-school experience of toxic parenting will simply consolidate the damage (including brain damage) that has already been done. Some children, however, will have had a good-enough (perhaps even excellent) infancy, only to find themselves, for whatever reason, confronted by a severe emotional abuse and neglect experience during the toddler and pre-school years. For these children, there will be a colossal anomic shock. Whether a new experience or just more of the same, there will be an identifiable range of ways in which the harm is expressed.

To avoid repetition, I shall highlight only some of those expressions characteristic of the toddler and pre-school years. Physically, the emotionally abused and neglected pre-schooler is likely to have an unsatisfying relationship with their own body, which it will be difficult for them to value, understand, or control. Difficult to value because nobody is telling them that it is attractive or that it needs to be cared for. Difficult to understand because nobody is helping them to interpret its signals. Difficult to control because its inherent tendency towards competence is either unrewarded or positively punished. The emotionally abused and neglected pre-schooler may have problems with bowel and bladder control. If the care is indifferent, toilet-training may be delayed. If the care is hostile or unpredictable, the whole business may be associated with anxiety and/or disgust. The child may be clumsy, accident-prone, fidgety, or unnervingly still.

This, of course, is the period in a child's life when their horizons are radically extended as a result of the development of language and play. Every proud parent or carer welcomes and encourages the song without words that is the precursor of language. However, the efforts of the neglected child to speak are met with indifference, or at best with inconsistent and limited encouragement, while the emotionally abused child might even be punished for speaking, or at least for saying the wrong thing. Of course language does not simply express thought and feeling, it is constitutive of both – if I do not develop language I do not get to think or feel properly. Similarly with play. Play is the child's laboratory, theatre, stadium, church and therapy. In play, the child finds out about the world, experiments with different roles, learns to compete and co-operate with their fellows, explores the meaning of life, and works through jagged and difficult experiences. If the child's inherent hunger for play is unsatisfied, their efforts in all these essential psychological and social tasks are thwarted. Without language and play, a child's capacity to learn is seriously hobbled.

Meanwhile, the damage to the child's capacity to form or to maintain secure attachments continues unabated. While the attachment process begins from birth, it is commonly accepted that the period between 6 months and 3 years is a critical one for the development of the capacity to make secure attachments. This vital aspect of successful human experience, so essential that John Bowlby[26] compared it to the body's need for vitamins and protein, is at risk of terminal damage for the child who experiences toxic parenting during the pre-school years. Attachment theorists rightly draw attention to the development of insecure attachment styles – the ambivalent, the avoidant, and the disorganised; the child who 'ups the ante' and screams and shouts for recognition and validation; the child who retreats into their shell to become, in the words of Simon and Garfunkel, 'a rock, …an island'; and the child who is, quite simply, all over the place emotionally. Emotionally abused and neglected pre-schoolers may be aggressive, withdrawn, or both by turns. They may be indiscriminate in their search for affection and/or attention. They may seek to comfort themselves by means of rocking, head-banging, and/or compulsive masturbation. Meanwhile, they may have terrible trouble with their peers. Not only may their poor self-care skills immediately alienate them from their peers, but they are likely to have very poor negotiating skills, and to be very bad at turn-taking.

PRIMARY SCHOOL

The experience of nursery and/or primary school is one replete with challenges and opportunities. All good-enough parents and carers go to great lengths to prepare their children for what is inescapably a crisis, albeit a crisis that is both essential and productive. For the emotionally abused and neglected child, who has already in all likelihood been dis-prepared for the experience in some (or all) the ways described, the crisis is likely to be nine parts threat and only one part opportunity – that is if the child even attends. Poor school attendance amongst primary school children is (in my view) almost diagnostic of neglect. Parents may keep their children off school for various, more or less understandable, reasons, and the children themselves may have their own reasons for wanting to stay at home. However, the primary school child who does not attend regularly and in good time is a child whose future is already beginning to look very bleak.

Even when she or he does attend school, the emotionally abused and neglected child will experience considerable difficulty finding their place in this wider and more challenging world. Most of the problems mentioned so far will still feature but there is more. Some emotionally abused and neglected children will (at a certain level) thrive at school. For one thing, they may encounter peers and adults who offer them something that they have either never had at all or only had fitfully at home. For another, it might be that immersion in schoolwork offers a huge and welcome distraction from the problems that beset the child at home. However, for many emotionally abused and neglected children, primary school is just another domain in which to fail – academically, emotionally, and socially. In addition to the damage already described, the emotionally abused and neglected primary school child may find it almost impossible to concentrate because home has provided so little in the way of routine, especially those routines that have to do with eating and sleeping.

In addition, the peer group may be a source of terror to the emotionally abused and neglected child. How frequently do you hear it said that such and such a child is excellent in the one-to-one with an adult but hopeless with peers and especially when two or three peers are gathered together? This is not hard to understand. One of the greatest challenges of every childhood is the transition from the asymmetrical world of parent–child relationships to the symmetrical world of peer–peer relationships. In the former, the parent normally gives without expecting much (if anything) in return. This is what we mean by unconditional love. In the latter, the accent is on trading. Peers generally expect a return on their investment, else they will take their stock elsewhere. Parents give, peers trade. It is very much harder to trade if you have never been given, so the emotionally abused and neglected child seeks out at school the asymmetrical relationship with the adult and avoids (or messes up) the symmetrical relationship with other children. Unfortunately, the target adult, who may or may not be a teacher, will probably have neither the time nor the capacity to satisfy the insatiable hunger of the emotionally abused and neglected child, at least not without real unfairness to the other children for whom they are responsible, so that a dreadful home experience is compounded by a non-reparative experience at school.

SECONDARY SCHOOL

By now, the emotionally abused and neglected child is well and truly learning to fail. For every child who compensates at school for their sense of failure and unhappiness at home, there must be hundreds who feel a comprehensive sense of failure in both domains. Many of the children have, by this time, effectively dropped out of school altogether. Others are there only in the flesh. The secondary school child may be completely withdrawn, or they may express their intense alienation through downright anti-social, criminal, even dangerous behaviour. The hunger to belong, to count for something, is basic to our nature. If we can not belong in one group, we will withdraw, or we will seek to belong to another. If we can not belong to a group in one way, we will belong in another way. The child may well be tempted either to establish and dominate their own sub-group, which may be at odds with what they see as 'the establishment', or they may be prepared to pay an exorbitant price for admission to somebody else's sub-group as an unthinkingly obedient lieutenant or general dogsbody. Such children are not learning to be independent but to be counter-dependent, which is a very different thing.

STATISTICS

As with so many politically charged subjects, one has to be careful with official statistics. Any interpretation of the figures contained in the following tables should bear in mind at least three possible distortions. First, there have been changes recently in the guidance given by central government concerning the categorisation of child abuse. Second, local government star-chasing may have resulted in a distortion downwards of the extent of actual child abuse. Third, the use of the Child Protection Register (and its successor) is almost certainly uneven across the country. That said, the figures do suggest some interesting recent trends.

Table 1 provides information about children registered on 31 March for the years between 1997–2003, gleaned from the DCFS website. Note that, year-on-year, there are far more registrations under the category of neglect than under any other category, and that for the most part there are fewer registrations under the category of emotional abuse than under any other category, the one exception being 2001, when there were slightly more emotional than sexual abuse registrations. That there were so relatively few emotional abuse registrations during this period should come as no surprise. In a study of 94 children registered under this category, published by BASPCAN in 2001, Glaser et al.[27] noted that the length of time between the first report of concern to Social Services and the date of registration ranged from 8 months to 14 years and 8 months, the mean being 4.06 years. A small statistic with a big significance.

Table 2, however, which deals with children subject to a child protection plan on 31 March each year between 2003 and 2007 gleaned from the DCSF website, shows a significant change. Note the slight increase in the number of

Table 1 Number of children on the Child Protection Register at 31 March in the years 1997–2003

	1997	1998	1999	2000	2001	2002	2003
Total	32,400	31,600	31,900	30,300	26,800	25,700	26,600
Neglect	**12,200**	**13,000**	**13,900**	**14,000**	**12,900**	**10,100**	**10,600**
Physical	10,900	9900	9100	8700	7300	4200	4300
Sexual	7400	6700	6600	5600	4500	4500	5000
Emotional	**5000**	**5200**	**5400**	**5500**	**4800**	**2800**	**2700**
Other	600	500	950	630	500	4100	4400

Table 2 Number of children subject to a child protection plan at 31 March in the years 2003–2007

	2003	2004	2005	2006	2007
Neglect	10,600	11,000	11,400	11,800	12,500
Physical	4300	4100	3900	3600	3500
Sexual	2700	2500	2400	2300	2000
Emotional	5000	5100	5200	6000	7100
Mixed	4000	3600	3000	2700	2700
Total	26,600	26,300	25,900	26,400	27,800

neglected children, and the quite significant increase in the number of emotionally abused children. Both increases are almost certainly related to the state's increasing acknowledgement of the emotional damage done to children by drug and alcohol misuse and by domestic violence. Sadly, but perhaps inevitably, the enormous damage inflicted upon children by litigious parents in private law disputes will not be reflected in these statistics. Most such children are untouched by the formal child protection system, in spite of the serious and chronic harm and distress involved. Sometimes, here it is the individual parent who is inflicting the harm. More often, it is what is happening between parents that produces the toxin.

THE SOIL IN WHICH EMOTIONAL ABUSE AND NEGLECT THRIVES

It is not difficult to describe the soil in which emotional abuse and neglect thrives, its interacting elements will be well known to all readers. I have deliberately used the metaphor of 'soil' so as to avoid an over-simplistic and mechanical idea about cause and effect.

Poverty and social exclusion

Poverty and social exclusion do not directly cause emotional abuse and neglect. Most poor parents and carers do an admirable best with the little that is available to them. Conversely, there are wealthy parents and carers who could give lessons to their poorer fellow citizens in how not to bring up children. Nevertheless, for reasons that hardly need to be rehearsed here, to be poor is to be vulnerable on just about every front, so that the task of rearing children is that much harder. It is surely not surprising that the vast majority of emotional abuse and neglect registrations concern children from the poorest families.

Early parenthood and large families

Young parents and carers are not necessarily less competent than their elders, and most large families are as loving as their smaller peer-families. Even so, early parenthood carries its own challenges. If young parents and carers are unprepared or unsupported, they may buckle under the strain. If they have many children over a relatively short period, they may find it very difficult to spread themselves around or keep control.

Domestic violence

Three-quarters of a million children each year in England and Wales suffer because of domestic violence. One in four reported violent crimes is domestic. Something like 80% of domestic assaults are not reported to the police. One in five murder victims is a woman killed by her current or former partner and more than half child protection cases include an element of domestic violence towards the mother.

Substance misuse

It is a commonplace that one can sustain a drug or alcohol habit and provide good-enough care for children. However, common sense indicates that an out-of-control habit will seriously compromise parenting (and just about every other important function as well). Of course, it is not just the immediate and toxic effects on the carer and the child of the substance. Chaotic substance misuse usually entails significant criminality, the misdirection of household income, a serious skewing of priorities with respect to routine and attention, and all too often a degree of violence and conflict as well. Children reared in environments of this kind are, in my view, ineluctably emotionally abused and neglected children, unless there is somebody in the kinship system who is able and willing to take the strain of caring on a more or less full-time basis.

Family breakdown

More than a third of children experience family breakdown. The vast majority of those children come nowhere near the child protection system, nor do I suggest that they should. However, they are an unsung group of children who, for a time at least, often experience emotional abuse and neglect, as their distressed and pre-occupied parents cope with their own sense of abandonment, guilt and betrayal. In most cases, after a period of intense distress, the parents concerned find a way of dealing with each other and their focus returns to their children. Most children, in turn, recover from the crisis without long-term damage, but this is not the case for all children. Witness those families which are dead but will not lie down, those parents who fight with each other for years in the courts, using the children as weapons, struggling endlessly about money, residence, contact and a variety of specific issues, most of which are distressingly beside the point.

Physical illness and disability

Here I must be very clear. There are, of course, ill and disabled parents and carers who neglect and emotionally abuse their children in just the same way as other parents and carers. It is important not to be sentimental, but most do nothing of the kind. Such gaps as there may be in the lives of children with ill or disabled parents or carers generally derive not from the carers themselves but from serious system failures – the barriers that a civilised society would long since have removed, and the absence of client-centred personal social services such as might level the playing-field for disabled carers.

Mental disorder

Many carers with mental health problems manage to raise happy and productive children. Most children with a mentally ill parent do not need to be rescued, though they often do need a bit of help and counselling. It is, of course, very much harder if both parents are mentally ill, harder still if that illness takes certain forms – paranoid schizophrenia, obsessive compulsive disorder, psychotic depression, for example. Perhaps the most difficult circumstance is the child who is being looked after by a carer with some kind of serious personality disorder. In addition to the diagnostic chaos that may surround such a carer, there will often be the usual unseemly struggle between the agencies as to who is and who is not responsible for providing help.

Learning difficulties

Yet again, I must note that adults with learning difficulties often rear happy and productive children. Yet again, it is important not to be sentimental; there are degrees and forms of learning difficulty that will make it very hard for an adult satisfactorily to meet some of the most basic needs of a child. This is nobody's fault, but emotional abuse and neglect is not necessarily anybody's fault or responsibility. Here is another area in which system responsibilities are very important.

Pre-occupation

This is a very general category. Pre-occupation is a feature of most of the above elements in the soil of emotional abuse and neglect, but those elements do not exhaust what I mean by pre-occupation. We live in a very stressful and competitive society, a society in which it is increasingly deemed necessary for both parents to work, a society in which nuclear families are increasingly unmoored from the wider kinship system, a society which is increasingly atomised and individualised. In such a society, children are likely to miss out on simple things like time and attention, however materially comfortable their parents may be. In years to come, I expect that the well-heeled emotionally abused and neglected child will attract increasing attention from the relevant systems.

LONG-TERM EFFECTS OF EMOTIONAL ABUSE AND NEGLECT

Many (perhaps even most) children who have experienced significant emotional abuse and neglect grow up determined to make a go of their lives and to ensure that their own children do not experience what they have experienced themselves. Some do not, and it is not difficult to set out the futures of those children who are, for one reason or another, unable to overcome their experience of emotional abuse and neglect. Basically, there are three kinds of morbid outcome. There are those adults who take it out on themselves, those who take it out on other people, and those who do both. These three morbid outcomes may be the consequence of a macabre interaction between neurophysiological, psychological, and social factors.

Those who take it out on themselves may develop a range of mental health problems, such as chronic anxiety, depression, and a general personal incapacity. They may develop serious sexual dysfunction. They may resort to substance misuse. They may develop eating and sleeping disorders.

Those who take it out on other people may become anti-social. They may become habitual criminals. They may become violent and abusive towards both adults and children. They may develop intractable problems with respect to intimacy and separation. In particular, they may have a frightening incapacity for empathy.

All of which significantly increases the chances, to adapt Philip Larkin, of man's handing on misery to man.[28]

WHY DO PROFESSIONALS SO OFTEN FAIL EMOTIONALLY ABUSED AND NEGLECTED CHILDREN?

That professionals and their agencies do fail emotional abuse and neglect children is beyond doubt. A cursory reading of the inquiry reports from Maria Colwell[29] to Victoria Climbié[30] would make this abundantly clear. Nor are the connected reasons hard to discern.

Insufficient resources

Emotional abuse and neglect work is time, labour, and resource intensive. Emotional abuse and neglect is a state rather than an event. It is not like a physical injury, which can be often be identified and diagnosed quickly.

Organisational problems

To say that we live in times of change is to state the obvious, but it is true. The shape and structure of health and social care are in a state of continual change. Indeed, no 'wannabe' manager who did not promise change would be appointed, and no 'wannabe' politician who did not threaten change would be elected. There is a managerial and political vocabulary out there that stresses progress, change, and moving forward (whatever that may mean). And the successful manager and politician will be one who is able to accomplish change, to incite the workforce to change, and to isolate and discredit sceptics, who will be branded as out-of-time, dinosaurs, reactionaries, or pitiful souls who are threatened by change, and who live in the past rather than in 'The Now'. Whatever the advantages of this 'dynamic' approach to the personal social services may be, there is a downside. An increasingly unstable workforce (at all levels), a disconnection between the agencies and the communities they are supposed to serve. An increasing reliance upon peripatetic staff. The development of memory-free, short-term projects whose staff, however skilled, well qualified and intentioned, have children of their own to feed at the end of the 3 years' funding. None of this is well adapted to emotional abuse and neglect work. Just one example. I have personal experience of a case in which a child had 10 social workers during Care Proceedings. Ten key workers in one set of public law proceedings is probably very unusual, frequent changes of social worker are not. Social workers spend a smaller proportion of their time actually working with families than they did even 10 years ago. Incidentally, I am told that this is also the case with health visitors, and it is certainly the case with probation officers. It is hard to see how quality work can be done in the field of emotional abuse and neglect in a climate such as this.

Poor training and supervision

Inquiry after inquiry has commented upon how poorly equipped essential staff often are in the field of child protection work in general, and they have frequently pointed out how poor supervision has contributed to the death of a child. As long ago as 1985, the Beckford Report reminded us of the four objectives of social work supervision in child protection:[31]

1. *To ensure that the social worker has the knowledge and skills to carry out his or her task.*

2. *To monitor the activities of the social worker.*

3. *To be aware of the attitudes of the social worker towards the case and to correct, if necessary, the way in which they affect handling of the case.*

4. *To support the social worker both practically and emotionally.*

These objectives can be easily extended to the other sectors of the child protection system. Otherwise, I stress here just one thing – the importance of supervisory continuity, especially in a world in which staff turnover is high and staff retention such a challenge.

Burn-out, tolerance, and habituation

Emotional abuse and neglect is high-stress work. Done properly, it involves a great deal of face-to-face contact with carers and children over a long period. That contact involves confrontation as well as sympathy, stick as well as carrot. The workers concerned regularly face anger, abuse, indifference, sometimes even violence. Small wonder that many burn out. Burn-out is a faceted phenomenon. One thing that happens to over-burdened staff is that their perceptions are altered in the face of continual stress. There is a kind of cognitive dissonance at work. If your entire caseload consists of emotionally abused and neglected children and their families you begin to compare the suffering children and young people not with what you would expect of a 'normal' child, but with each other. This child is not as miserable as that one. This family is a bit better than that one. It is but a small step now to imagining that the less miserable child is not miserable, that the bit better coping family is not causing harm at all. Such a shift in perception is not an accident. It is a cognitive distortion the effect of which is to provide us with false re-assurance. Have you noticed from the inquiries how often it is that the civilians see what the professionals have missed even though it has been in front of their eyes all along? It is surely no accident, for example, that the two people who emerged with their integrity unscathed in the Laming Report were the unregistered child minder who took Victoria Climbié to the Central Middlesex Hospital on 14 July 1999, and the minicab-driver who took the child to the Tottenham Ambulance Station on the last night of her life, 24 February 2000.

Professional guilt and identification with parents

Professional guilt is wide-spread, why wouldn't it be? Most workers in this field have reasonable incomes and can pay the bills. Most of the families that we police have pitiful incomes and their bills are a source of constant anxiety. Most decent people with a reasonable income will think twice before drawing attention to the failings of carers without one. Sometimes, we will carry that diffidence to great lengths, so that our powerless sense of identification with the parent may blind us to the plight of the child.

Fear

Fear of parents, fear of consequences, fear of come-back – and we are right to be afraid. Afraid that we will be abused, perhaps even assaulted. Afraid that if we do intervene we will open a Pandora's box of consequences that may cause more harm to the child and their parents than the emotional abuse and neglect that we think we have identified. Afraid that, if we do not intervene, we shall be held to public account. All these things can hobble our confidence in a very difficult and challenging area of work.

CONCLUDING REMARKS

Emotionallly abused and neglected families can often be turned round. There are two relevant sets of factors here – those that have to do with the family, and those that have to do with the child welfare system. The future looks good for families in which: (i) relationships are generally affectionate; (ii) the adults are able to take at least some responsibility for the emotional abuse and neglect and for the changes that are necessary to put things right; (iii) the family has steadfast and clear-sighted informal support from wider kin, friends and neighbours; (iv) there are no major stressors in the offing; (v) there is no violence; (vi) substance use is at least under control; and (vii) it is possible for the adults to establish collaborative relationships with the helping agencies.

However, it would be wrong to gaze only at the families themselves, else we are merely biographers. I have already said that work in emotional abuse and neglect is time-, skill-, and resource-hungry work. If we are to make a difference, there are agency factors to be taken into account. The future looks good for families when the agency culture meets the following standards: (i) when there is an optimistic agency culture about prevention; (ii) when there is a range of resources (including well-staffed family centres); (iii) when there is a skilled, experienced, confident and stable workforce; (iv) when there is consistent, empowering supervision; (v) when there is a collaborative professional culture so that no agency is left to go it alone; and (vi) when there is a degree of organisational stability. You do the maths!

Key points for clinical practice

- Emotional abuse and neglect are at the heart of child abuse. They absolutely are not the lesser forms of child abuse. Even if they do not often lead to death, and sometimes they do especially in the case of very young children, they can radically damage a child's brain, mind, and heart, which is why I sometimes speak of toxic parenting.

- Emotional abuse and neglect may be conceptually distinct, and one may exist without the other. In most cases, they co-exist, which is why I speak of emotional abuse and neglect or toxic parenting.

- Emotional abuse and neglect is a state rather than an event. You will occasionally come across single episodes of such drama and intensity that it will be right to think of these as emotional abuse and neglect. For the most part, emotional abuse and neglect is an awful accumulation of small sins of omission and commission, which is one of the reasons it often goes undetected until it is almost too late to do anything about it.

(continued)

Key points for clinical practice *(continued)*

- Severe emotional abuse and neglect may begin as early as conception; if it continues into early infancy and beyond, the likelihood is that the child will sustain serious damage. The damage to the child's brain and to their capacity to make and sustain secure attachments are particularly worrying.

- Emotional abuse and neglect is the consequence, not simply of hostile or indifferent parenting, but also of incompetent parenting. It occurs whenever parents or carers are unprepared for, or are long-term distracted from, the business of caring for the child concerned.

- Emotional abuse and neglect is almost always a central feature in those cases which are labelled child abuse and which involve local authorities, child protection plans, and public law proceedings. It is all too often a central feature in cases which never come anywhere near the formal child protection system. For example, in intractable and bitter private law disputes about residence and contact, in child and adolescent mental health referrals, and in cases involving the juvenile justice system.

- Proper identification of emotional abuse and neglect will almost always be an inter-disciplinary and multi-agency. No one sector of the child welfare system has a monopoly of knowledge and experience in this area.

- Proper identification of emotional abuse and neglect will call upon a practitioner's imagination and empathy as much as (if not more than) their clinical knowledge and experience. Indeed, there is some evidence that professionals may be less likely than civilians to recognise what is in front of their eyes. Always the question should be: 'What must it be like to be this child in these circumstances, cared for in this way, by these people?'

- Paradoxically, while early and energetic intervention in emotional abuse and neglect is almost certainly the best way to alleviate the plight of the children concerned, it is precisely in the case of emotional abuse and neglect that intervention is likely to be late, uncoordinated and clumsy.

- There are features of the contemporary child welfare, health, and family justice systems that make them very poorly equipped to deal with emotional abuse and neglect. Not least the rapid turnover of staff, the pace and style of organisational change, the pre-occupation of all the sectors with thresholds, boundaries and key performance indicators, and the documented chronic incapacity of all the sectors to work together to protect children.

- In the care of children, it is probably always important to take a whole-child approach. Where emotional abuse and neglect is concerned, nothing less than a whole-child approach will do.

Bibliography

1. Miller A. *The Drama of Being a Child*. Virago, 1987; and *Thou Shalt Not Be Aware: Society's Betrayal of The Child*, 2nd edn. Pluto Press, 1998.
2. Garbarino, Guttmann, Seeley. *The Psychologically Battered Child: Strategies for Identification and Intervention*. Jossey Bass, 1986.
3. *Journal of Social Welfare Law* 1988.
4. Bettelheim B. *The Empty Fortress: Infantile Autism and the Birth of the Self*. Free Press, 1967.
5. Laing RD, Esterson A. *Sanity, Madness and the Family*. Tavistock, 1964.
6. O'Hagan K. *Emotional and Psychological Abuse of Children*. Open University, 1993.
7. Iwaniec D. *The Emotionally Abused and Neglected Child*, 2nd edn. Wiley Blackwell, 2006; and *Children Who Fail to Thrive: A Practice Guide*. Wiley, 2004.
8. Garbarino, Guttmann, Seeley. *The Psychologically Battered Child: Strategies for Identification and Intervention*. Jossey Bass, 1986; 9–10.
9. *Ibid*. page 7.
10. *Ibid*. page 44.
11. *Ibid*. page 8.
12. Glaser D. Emotional abuse and neglect (psychological maltreatment): a conceptual framework. In: *Child Abuse & Neglect*, vol. 26. 2002; 697–714.
13. Garbarino, Guttmann, Seeley. *The Psychologically Battered Child: Strategies for Identification and Intervention*. Jossey Bass, 1986; 45.
14. The concept of the 'identified patient' derives from the work of Virginia Satir. See especially her *Conjoint Family Therapy*, 3rd edn. Science and Behavior Books, 1983.
15. Department of Health. *Child Protection: Messages from Research*. London: HMSO, 1995; 19.
16. See: Waterhouse, Pitcairn, McGhee, Sullivan *Evaluating Parenting in Child Physical Abuse*. Jessica Kingsley, 1993.
17. Department for Children, Schools and Families. *Safeguarding Children in whom Illness is Fabricated or Induced*. 2008.
18. Gardner, Richard A. *The Parental Alienation Syndrome: A Guide for Mental Health and Legal Professionals*, 2nd edn. Creative Therapeutics, 1998; and Department for Children, Schools and Families. *Safeguarding Children in whom Illness is Fabricated or Induced*. 2008.
19. Freud A. *The Ego and The Mechanisms of Defence*. Hogarth Press and the Institute of Psycho-Analysis, 1968.
20. S31(9).
21. See, for example: Streissguth A. *Fetal Alcohol Syndrome: A Guide for Families and Communities*. Brookes 1997; Janov A. *The Biology of Love*. Prometheus Books, 2000; Gerhardt S. *Why Love Matters: How Affection Shapes a Baby's Brain*. Routledge, 2004; James O. *The F*** You Up: How To Survive Family Life*, revised edn. Bloomsbury, 2007; Karr-Morse R, Wiley M. *Ghosts from the Nursery*. New York: Atlantic Monthly Press, 1997.
22. *Op. Cit*. page 167.
23. Deacon T. *The Symbolic Species*. London: Penguin, 1997.
24. LeDoux J. *Synaptic Self: How Our Brains Become Who We Are*. London: Penguin, 2002.
25. Gerhardt S. *Why Love Matters: How Affection Shapes a Baby's Brain*. Routledge, 2004.
26. Bowlby J. *Attachment*. Hogarth Press and the Institute of Psycho-Analysis, 1969.
27. Glaser D, Prior V, Lynch MA. *Emotional Abuse and Emotional Neglect: Antecedents, Operational Definitions and Consequences [BASPCAN]*. 2001, iii.
28. Larkin P. *Collected Poems*. Marvell Press and Faber & Faber, 1988; 180.
29. Secretary of State for Social Services. *Report of the Inquiry into the Care and Supervision Provided in Relation to Maria Colwell*. London: HMSO, 1974.
30. Lord Laming. *The Victoria Climbié Inquiry*. London: Stationery Office, 2003.
31. London Borough of Brent. *A Child In Trust: The Report of the Panel of Inquiry into the Circumstances Surrounding the Death of Jasmine Beckford*. 1985; chapter 21.

Brook Belay Peter F. Belamarich

5

Statin therapy in children

With the progression of the obesity epidemic and type 2 diabetes mellitus, prior trends in diminishing the burden of cardiovascular disease on a global level are likely to be negated.

The 3-hydroxy-3-methylglutaryl coenzyme A reductase inhibitors (statins), first developed in Japan in 1973 and launched in 1987 in the US with the use of lovastatin, have been markedly effective in the prevention of myocardial infarction in high-risk adults and have become the cornerstone of therapy in cardiovascular disease prevention. However, their use in children is based on a chain of evidence that links established cardiovascular risk factors in childhood to pre-morbid pathological changes found in autopsies of high-risk adolescents. This has led to a motivation to prevent the progression of atherosclerotic plaque in its earliest stages. Central to this motivation is the hypothesis that statins started before the formation of significant burden of atherosclerotic plaque will have a greater benefit than seen when they are begun in adulthood.

Direct evidence that statins, when begun in childhood, can prevent cardiovascular events in childhood or adulthood is lacking. Consequently, many important questions remain. Paediatricians have a special obligation to master the safe use of statins because they are treating asymptomatic individuals who are taking these drugs in advance of any discernible clinical disease. To date, the primary indication for statin therapy in children has been limited to children with severe dyslipidaemia resulting from heterozygous

Brook Belay MD (for correspondence)
Assistant Professor of Pediatrics, Department of Pediatrics, Temple University School of Medicine, Philadelphia, PA 19140, USA.
E-mail: brook.belay@tuhs.temple.edu

Peter F. Belamarich MD
Director, Pediatric Ambulatory Subspecialty Practices, Associate Professor of Clinical Pediatrics, Department of Pediatrics, Albert Einstein College of Medicine, Children's Hospital at Montefiore, Bronx, NY 10467, USA

familial hypercholesterolaemia, but their wider use in children suffering from other conditions associated with cardiovascular disease in early adulthood is growing.

This chapter reviews new insights in the cholesterol hypothesis relevant to statin use. Then, the previous experience with statin therapy in both adults and children is reviewed with a special focus on safety considerations. The use of surrogate markers of disease and outcomes, including imaging studies, is also addressed.

CHOLESTEROL HYPOTHESIS, ATHEROSCLEROSIS AND STATINS

PATHOPHYSIOLOGY

A complete review of the cholesterol hypothesis and the mechanisms involved in atherosclerosis is beyond the scope of this chapter, but has been appraised elsewhere recently.[1] A brief review, however, would highlight that the pathophysiological process involves not simply an elevation in low-density lipoprotein cholesterol levels resulting in sub-endothelial lipid accretion, but a complex interplay between inflammatory and growth-regulating molecules and multiple cell types. Oxidised low-density lipoprotein cholesterol particles accumulate in macrophages (foam cells), which adhere to and accumulate beneath the arterial endothelial layer. The elaboration of chemokines that attract and activate circulating monocytes and T-lymphocytes to the region, are part of an immune response that is self-amplifying. Endothelial and smooth muscle cells also exhibit altered functioning, including reduced expression of the vasodilatory nitric oxide. Eventually, at a gross level, fatty streaks progress to fibrous plaques and then to more complex advanced plaques that are heterogeneous collections of lipid, and cells covered by a tenuous collagen matrix that forms a fibrous cap. A large proportion of complex plaques grow centrifugally and do not occlude the vascular lumen, a phenomenon known as the Glagov hypothesis,[2] and yet are capable of precipitating a thrombotic occlusion. Infarctions can be precipitated by an erosion or disruption of the cap, a spontaneous rupture of the plaque, or a haemorrhage into the plaque causing disruption; all of these mechanisms can precipitate platelet adhesion, activation and thrombus formation. The size and reversibility of the luminal thrombus and the extent of collateral circulation dictate the extent of the ischaemic insult to the myocardium.

Statins given at doses that are associated with a substantially reduced cardiovascular disease risk do not consistently cause a significant regression of plaque volume.[3] As a consequence, it is thought that statins may act by modulating the risk of erosion, disruption and/or haemorrhage. That is, statins may work by a qualitative transformation of high-risk plaque into a lower risk state. This is theoretically important because the prescription of statins to paediatric or adolescent patients is intended to prevent the formation or progression of plaque rather than reduce the intrinsic risk of rupture.

PHARMACOLOGY OF STATINS

Currently, there are seven statins available for clinical use world-wide (Table 1), although their licensure varies by location especially for children. For

Table 1 Statins in use world-wide

Name[a]	Age range (years)	Dose range[b] (mg/day)	Metabolic pathway
Atorvastatin[c] (Lipitor®, Atorlip®)	10–17	10–20	CYP3A3/4 substrate; CYP3A4 inhibitor
Fluvastatin[c] (Lescol®, Canef®)	10-16	20-40	CYP2C9 substrate
Lovastatin[c] (Mevacor®, Altacor®)	10–17	10–40	CYP3A3/4 substrate
Pitavastatin (Itavastatin®)			CYP2C9 substrate (minimal)
Pravastatin[c] (Pravachol®, Lipostat®)	8–13 14-18	20 40	CYP3A3/4 substrate; CYP3A4, CYP2C8/9 (minimal), CYP2D6 inhibitor
Rosuvastatin (Crestor®)			CYP2C9 substrate (minimal)
Simvastatin[c] (Zocor®)	10–17	10–40	CYP3A3/4 substrate

A listing of various statins, their metabolic pathway and appropriate paediatric age groups of use and dosages is shown. Where appropriate, paediatric age groups for which statins have been approved are displayed. A starting dose is provided with dose adjustment changes possible up to a maximum. For specific prescribing information see drug manuals.
[a]International non-proprietary names are listed with selected trade names in parentheses.
[b]The listed doses have equivalent degrees of lipid-reduction at the indicated starting dose.
[c]Approved for use in the US in children.
Reproduced with permission from Belay et al.[27] © 2007 by the American Academy of Pediatrics.

example, in the US, five of these statins are licensed for use in children.

All statins inhibit the critical step in cholesterol biosynthesis – the enzyme 3-hydroxy-3-methylglutaryl coenzyme A reductase (Fig. 1). This inhibition leads to an increase in expression low-density lipoprotein cholesterol receptors on the hepatic cellular surface and consequently uptake of low-density lipoprotein cholesterol from the circulation. This is the predominant mechanism by which the plasma concentration of low-density lipoprotein-cholesterol is reduced; generally, statins lower plasma concentrations of low-density lipoprotein cholesterol by 25–45%.[4,5] Their use is also associated with mild, but significant, elevations in high-density-lipoprotein cholesterol of 1–6%.[5] Statins do not lower plasma triglyceride levels and, therefore, are not indicated for the treatment of isolated hypertriglycerideaemia.

All statins are metabolised by the hepatic cytochrome P450 system (Table 1). This makes statins susceptible to competitive inhibition at this level, which may increase the risk of statin-related toxicities, including myopathy, in particular. Statins vary in their lipophilicity; pitavastatin and pravastatin are the least lipophilic and lovastatin and simvastatin are amongst the most lipophilic drugs. Although all statins inhibit the reductase enzyme, their physiochemical and pharmacological properties vary significantly. It is not known currently whether these differences confer a relative benefit or risk for children or adolescents, but this is an area that deserves further deliberate study and attention as data accumulate.

Concentrations of mevalonate intermediates downstream of the reductase enzyme are also affected by statins (Fig. 1) – namely, farnesyl pyrophosphate (FPP) and geranyl pyrophosphate (GPP). Consequently, the modification of regulatory pathways involved in cellular proliferation and immune responses may be altered with statin therapy. It has been hypothesised that this may represent an important mechanism by which statins exert anti-inflammatory and immune-modulatory effects on the atherosclerotic process. Furthermore, a direct reduction in T-lymphocyte cell membrane cholesterol rafts necessary for cellular signalling may be another mechanism by which statins affect inflammatory cascades in atherosclerosis.[6,7]

The pleiotropic effects of statins refer to those off-target effects of statins (*i.e.* not related to low density lipoprotein cholesterol reductions).[8] The mechanisms involved appear to be the non-cholesterol intermediates down-stream of 3-hydroxy-3-methylglutaryl coenzyme A reductase as outlined above. As such, reductions in lipid-based isoprenoids that are important in cellular signalling may be one mechanism of pleiotropy. Increased endothelial production of nitric oxide, an important vasodilator, has also been described with statin therapy. The relevance and contribution of these pleiotropic effects to disease outcomes in adults is still being defined and will be an important area to follow in paediatrics.

CLINICAL EFFECTS OF STATIN THERAPY

ADULT STATIN STUDIES

Amongst adults with a high risk for cardiovascular events. low density lipoprotein reductions are associated with a 26.6% reduction in any coronary heart disease related event.[4] Randomised clinical trials of statins have convincingly shown a linear correlation between the degree of lipid lowering in high-risk adults and the degree of reduction in cardiovascular disease rates. This link between lipid level reduction and cardiovascular outcomes has made low density lipoprotein cholesterol the traditional target of therapy. Some of these benefits of statin therapy have been attributed to their anti-inflammatory and immunomodulatory effects.[9]

The role of inflammation in the progress of atherosclerosis is also supported by studies that target individuals with elevations of high-sensitivity C-reactive protein. Reductions in high-sensitivity C-reactive protein correlate with reductions in cardiovascular disease rates.[10] Inclusion of such non-traditional risk factors also improves predictive value in cardiovascular risk assessment in adults treated with statins.[11] High-sensitivity C-reactive protein as a treatment target, however, has not been explored in children.

The effects of statin therapy on the progression of the atherosclerotic plaque have also been studied. Atherosclerotic plaques may remodel the vasculature by staying external to the lumen, as opposed to obstructing it. Imaging modalities such as intravascular ultrasonography have been important in understanding this process.[12] There is evidence that some statins have the ability to retard the progression of the atherosclerotic plaque. However, despite the clear benefits in cardiovascular outcomes with statin therapy, studies of the atherosclerotic lesions in treated adults show that these lesions

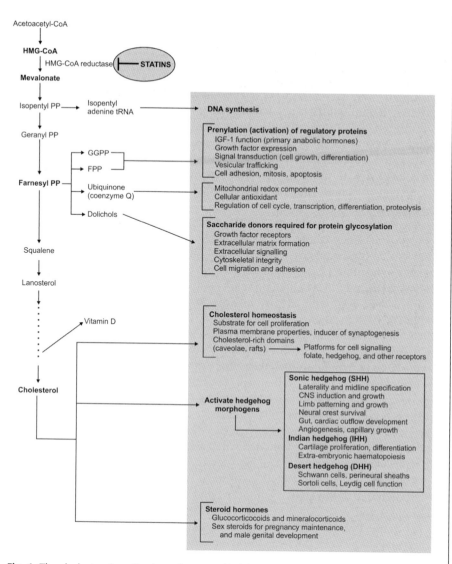

Fig. 1 The cholesterol synthesis pathway and inhibition by statins. A schematic of the cholesterol synthetic pathway depicting the rate determining step where statins inhibit 3-hydroxy-3-methylglutaryl coenzyme A reductase. Also shown are the full range of products downstream from the inhibited step that may be affected by statin therapy, including protein prenylation by farnesyl pyrophosphate (FPP) and geranylgeranyl pyrophosphate (GGPP). Reproduced from Edison and Muenke[36] © 2004 Wiley-Liss, Inc. Reprinted with permission of Wiley-Liss, Inc., a subsidiary of John Wiley & Sons, Inc.

either do not progress further or regress minimally in volume.[13] It appears that some patients simply benefit from stabilization of high-risk plaques.

In summary, adult statin studies provide valuable information on the efficacy of therapy for both major outcomes as well as surrogate markers of control over the atherosclerotic process. Imaging studies have enhanced understanding of the dynamic nature of the atherosclerotic plaque and how statin therapy may ameliorate cardiovascular disease.

SAFETY OF STATINS IN ADULTS

Information about statin safety derives from the very large cohort of adults who have been enrolled in randomised trials, from populations whose therapeutic course is recorded on electronic medical record databases and from post-marketing surveillance. Given the large numbers of adults enrolled in carefully monitored trials and subsequently treated, much is known about the adverse effects of statins: although generally well tolerated, they are not without their risks.[14] To date, the most significant adverse event associated with statins appears to be a spectrum of muscle involvement from myalgias unassociated with any laboratory changes to myopathy (defined as muscle complaints in conjunction with an elevation of creatine phosphokinase $\geq$ 10-times the upper limit of normal) to rhabdomyolysis associated with multi-organ failure and death in adults. Asymptomatic elevations in creatine phosphokinase are common.[14] Rhabdomyolysis requiring hospitalisation is a rare event – the number of individuals on statin monotherapy for 1 year needed to result in 1 case of rhabdomyolysis requiring hospitalisation has been estimated to be 1/23,000. Rhabdomyolysis appears to be a class and dose effect that has been seen with all currently available statin drugs. Cerivastatin was withdrawn from the market in the US because of an elevated risk of rhabdomyolysis noted in post-marketing surveillance.[15] Combination therapy with fibrates may increase the risk of such events.[16] This highlights the importance of maintaining vigilance for drug interactions.

Hepatotoxicity, defined as transient elevations in hepatic enzymes > 3-times the upper limit of normal on two consecutive measurements, may occur in ~1% of patients on statins.[14] The majority of these elevations are asymptomatic and liver damage is rare. Most hepatic enzyme elevations occur more than 90 days after initiation of therapy. There is evidence that aggressive therapy with higher doses of statins may increase the risk of hepatic enzyme elevation to ~3%.

Concerns that statins may be associated with an increased cancer risk and even cognitive decline have been raised and studies in large randomised trials and meta-analyses.[17] These concerns are balanced by a literature that suggests a neutral or even protective effect from statins on these same outcomes.[18,19] These questions have not been resolved definitively as of yet. Recent research has also focused on a statin effect on osteoclast activity, bone density and on the healing of fractures.[20]

Statins may be prescribed for either primary or secondary intervention, for example, for individuals who have never had a cardiovascular event, or in those who have previously had one, respectively. Statin studies conducted in adults as secondary prevention trials can undoubtedly be said to demonstrate the benefits of these drugs in reducing future cardiovascular events.

In contrast, the question of whether or not statins are effective in primary prevention has recently received critical attention.[21] It has been suggested that statins do not confer any benefit at the primary prevention level in adults.

Why is this observation important? From a public health perspective, the majority of the population of individuals for whom statin therapy would be indicated would fall under primary prevention. Most children and adolescents would fall in this category since they have never had a cardiovascular event. Lastly, if the benefits derived from statin therapy are related to their capacity to reduce the propensity of high-risk plaque to precipitate a luminal thrombus, it is possible that children whose plaques are at a much different stage of development might not benefit as much as would be predicted by the current chain of evidence. This is clearly an area that is highly important for paediatricians to follow as new information emerges especially since atherosclerosis is a continuum from childhood to adulthood and that therapy may be considered early on.[22]

SUMMARY OF PAEDIATRIC STATIN STUDIES

Statin therapy in paediatrics has resided not in the general paediatric population with clustered risk factors,[23] but in those children and adolescents with an inherited dyslipidaemia, heterozygous familial hypercholesterolaemia. Both in Europe and the US, studies of statins in children and adolescents and subsequent licensing of statins for paediatrics have focused on individuals with heterozygous familial hypercholesterolaemia. Individuals with this condition have one of over 700 mutations in the low-density lipoprotein cholesterol receptor that result in marked elevations of low density lipoprotein cholesterol. It is inherited as an autosomal co-dominant condition with quantitatively equal amounts of gene products from alleles contributed by each parent. The population prevalence is approximately 1:500 for heterozygotes and 1:1 million for homozygotes. Because of the large number of mutations, genetic testing is generally not clinically available. Consequently, several clinical working definitions for the diagnosis of heterozygous familial hypercholesterolaemia exist including: (i) marked elevations in low density lipoprotein cholesterol and/or total cholesterol measurements; (ii) a family history with 50% of first-degree relatives being affected (*i.e.* one parent and one grand-parent); (iii) evidence of early cardiovascular disease in first degree relatives; (iv) the presence of tendinous xanthomas; and (v) exclusion of causes of secondary dyslipidaemia. Generally, however, in the absence of any secondary causes and with the family history of dyslipidaemia, heterozygous familial hypercholesterolaemia can be diagnosed with low-density lipoprotein concentrations between 189–503 mg/dl (4.9–13.0 mmol/l) or a total cholesterol > 6.8 mmol/l.[24,25]

There is a markedly elevated risk of cardiovascular disease in early-to-mid-adulthood in this condition, in contrast to the homozygous form where cardiovascular events occur in childhood. However, the homozygous form is generally not responsive to statins because of the lack of functional low-density lipoprotein cholesterol receptors to be up-regulated.

Prior to the landmark lovastatin study in adolescent males with heterozygous familial hypercholesterolaemia (LAMS),[24] most statin trials were small in size and short in duration.[26] Statins are associated with major reductions in low-density lipoprotein cholesterol in the range of 30–50% that were not seen with drugs previously used to treat dyslipidaemia in these patients.[27] There is preliminary data from a prospective registry to suggest that statin therapy may reduce mortality risk in patients with heterozygous familial hypercholesterolaemia.[28]

Two studies involving surrogate measures of atherosclerosis have investigated the effects of statins on vascular function and morphology. de Jongh *et al.*[29] conducted a study assessing the ability of statins to reverse the early stages of endothelial dysfunction with flow-mediated dilatation in 50 children with heterozygous familial hypercholesterolaemia with simvastatin as compared to placebo. Simvastatin therapy was associated with improvements in flow-mediated dilatation of 4% and a 40% reduction in low-density lipoprotein cholesterol. Weigman *et al.*[30] conducted a randomised study investigating the efficacy of pravastatin in modulating carotid intima media thickness in paediatric patients with heterozygous familial hypercholesterolaemia. In this study, therapy was associated with a reduction in carotid thickness, as opposed to an increase in the placebo group.

Although the vast majority of the statin literature in paediatrics is in the field of familial hypercholesterolaemia, several studies have demonstrated marked reductions in low-density lipoprotein cholesterol with the use of statins in other high-risk groups of children including those with nephrotic syndrome, and kidney and heart transplants.[31-33] Hyperlipidaemia is hypothesised to be linked to chronic kidney disease via mechanisms involving oxidative stress and inflammation. Heart transplant recipients are at risk for accelerated atherosclerosis by way of graft vasculopathy, dyslipidaemia and pro-lipidaemic therapeutic regimens that include corticosteroids and drugs like tacrolimus. Treatment with statins has been associated with reduced rates of rejection at least in adult renal transplant recipients.[34]

One expert group has recently recommended the use of statins to prevent cardiovascular disease in children with high-risk conditions (*e.g.* transplant recipients, patients with diabetes mellitus type 1 and 2, patients with chronic kidney disease, and children with Kawasaki's disease).[35] Long-term data are needed to clarify the use of statins in these conditions.

SAFETY OF STATINS IN CHILDREN

The long-term safety of statins initiated in childhood is not addressed by the short-term studies done to date. Although longer-term data from adult studies is re-assuring, it does not answer the fundamental question of whether developing organisms exposed to statins for a potentially longer duration are susceptible to unique toxicities.

A recent meta-analysis did not report any significant differences in serious adverse effects in 476 children, 8–18 years of age, treated with various statins for 12–104 weeks (or ~2 years).[5] These studies have been re-assuring in that they have not shown any effects on growth and development in the short term. However, these studies, with only 476 patients on statins for 2 years, are underpowered to detect the presence of unique paediatric toxicities.

The utility and efficacy of routine laboratory monitoring in children on statins remains unexplored. Maintaining vigilance for use of other medications that may inhibit the cytochrome P-450 systems may minimise toxicity. Some of the more commonly used medications that inhibit these systems include macrolide antibiotics, antifungals, HIV-protease inhibitors, calcium channel blockers, and cyclosporine. Other medications induce the cytochrome system and may reduce serum statin levels (*e.g.* rifampin, carbamezapine and the barbiturates).

Finally, statins have been implicated in teratological changes and adverse birth outcomes in neonates whose mothers took statins during pregnancy.[36]

The pathophysiological mechanism appears to involve the lipophilic statins which can cross the placenta and inhibit cholesterol synthesis and sterol-dependent morphogens. Thus, statins should not be prescribed to adolescent females who could intentionally or unintentionally become pregnant.

THE FUTURE IN PAEDIATRIC ATHEROSCLEROSIS

As evidence and experience accumulate both with conditions that have an intrinsically increased risk of cardiovascular disease in childhood to adulthood, and with therapies that can effectively ameliorate that risk, the appropriate use and safety of drugs like statins will be clarified. Continued study and experience will elucidate the role of statins as recommended by the recent American Academy of Pediatrics policy on lipid screening. This policy recommends consideration of pharmacological therapy in the general paediatric population as young as 8 years of age with an elevated low-density lipoprotein cholesterol level and no other risk factors.[37]

As mentioned previously, recent guidelines in cardiovascular risk reduction in high-risk groups takes the first step in this direction by stratifying risk in different conditions, like kidney disease, diabetes mellitus types 1 and 2, transplantation, Kawasaki's disease and the inherited dyslipidaemias and making recommendations on evaluation and treatment.[35]

Similarly, the use of new imaging modalities to assess changes in vascular morphology and function will increase. The many new techniques in vascular imaging that are being developed hold promise in this regard.[38] What will remain crucial will be to determine which non-invasive modalities can capture and predict the complex phenomenon of cardiovascular risk.

Key points for clinical practice

- Currently, there is a consensus of expert opinion that statins be used for children with heterozygous familial hypercholesterolaemia or low-density lipoprotein cholesterol levels over 190 mg/dl (4.9 mmol/l).

No data have directly linked the treatment of statins in adolescents to cardiovascular outcomes. Therefore, this recommendation is based on a synthesis of evidence and expert opinion.

Most experts and practitioners agree that, when the setting is appropriate, statins should be introduced in the second decade of life.

There are many unanswered questions regarding the use of statins in cardiovascular prevention in paediatrics, including how to optimise the risk:benefit ratio for an individual patient.

Similarly, questions regarding safety of statins in children and adolescents including long-term and/or effects in the developing organism remain unanswered.

(continued)

Key points for clinical practice *(cont'd)*

- Because of safety concerns, physicians prescribing statins should be aware of their appropriate indications and potential drugs interactions.

- Likewise, pharmacists should especially be aware of potential interactions when a patient fills a prescription for a statin.

- Patients and their families should understand that, at this point, statin therapy is based on a chain of evidence and not evidence of direct effects on cardiovascular outcomes.

- Patients and their families should be educated about the benefits and risks associated with statin therapy and they should be advised on warning symptoms of possible adverse events such as muscle pain and abdominal pain and/or vomiting.

- Patients and their families should be advised to report any potential adverse events immediately to a healthcare provider. They should also have rapid access to their healthcare provider.

- Recommendations to use statins to prevent cardiovascular disease in children with other high-risk conditions in conjunction with hypercholesterolaemia has recently been broadened in the US.

- Newer imaging tools will have to be carefully assessed for their safety, feasibility and their ability to assess the rupture-risk of a plaque, a key issue in paediatrics.

References

1. Libby P. The molecular mechanisms of the thrombotic complications of atherosclerosis. *J Intern Med* 2008; **263**: 517–527.
2. Glagov S, Weisenberg E, Zarins CK, Stankunavicius R, Koletis GJ. Compensatory enlargement of the human atherosclerotic coronary arteries. *N Engl J Med* 1987; **316**: 1371–1375.
3. Ballantyne CM, Raichlen JS, Nicholls SJ et al. Effect of rosuvastatin therapy on coronary artery stenoses assessed by quantitative coronary angiography. A study to evaluate the effect of rosuvastatin on intravascular ultrasound-derived atheroma burden. *Circulation* 2008; **117**: 2458–2466.
4. Gould AL, Davies GM, Alemao E, Yin DD, Cook JR. Cholesterol reduction yields clinical benefits: meta-analysis including recent trials. *Clin Ther* 2007; **29**: 778–794.
5. Avis HJ, Vissers MN, Stein EA et al. A systematic review of and meta-analysis of statin therapy in children with familial hypercholesterolemia. *Arterioscler Thromb Vasc Biol* 2007; **27**: 1803–1810.
6. Ehrenstein MR, Jury EC, Mauri C. Statins for atherosclerosis – as good as it gets? *N Engl J Med* 2005; **352**: 73–75.
7. Dietzen DJ, Page KL, Tetzloff TA, Bohrer A, Turk J. Inhibition of 3-hydroxy-3-methylglutaryl coenzyme A (HMG CoA) reductase blunts factor VIIa / tissue factor and prothrombinase activities via effects on membrane phosphatidylserine. *Arterioscler Thromb Vasc Biol* 2007; **27**: 690–696.
8. Wang CY, Liu PY, Liao JK. Pleiotropic effects of statin therapy: molecular mechanisms and clinical results. *Trends Mol Med* 2008; **14**: 37–44.
9. Davidson MH. Clinical significance of statin pleiotropic effects: hypotheses versus evidence. *Circulation* 2005; **111**: 2280–2281.

10. Cannon CP, Braunwald E, McCabe CH *et al.* Intensive versus moderate lipid lowering with statins after acute coronary syndromes. *N Engl J Med* 2004; **350**: 1495–1504.

11. Danesh J, Wheeler JG, Hirschfield GM *et al.* C-reactive protein and other circulating factors of inflammation in the prediction of coronary heart disease. *N Engl J Med* 2004; **350**: 1387–1397.

12. Nash DT. Use of vascular ultrasound in clinical trials to evaluate new cardiovascular therapies. *J Natl Med Assoc* 2008; **100**: 222–229.

13. Nissen SE, Tuzcu EM, Schoenhagen P *et al.* Effect of intensive compared with moderate lipid-lowering therapy on progression of coronary atherosclerosis: a randomized controlled trial. *JAMA* 2004; **291**: 1071–1080.

14. Armitage J. The safety of statins in clinical practice. *Lancet* 2007; **370**: 1781–1790.

15. Furberg CD, Pitt B. Withdrawal of cerivastatin from the world market. *Curr Control Trials Cardiovasc Med* 2001; **2**: 205–207.

16. Graham DJ, Staffa JA, Shatin D *et al.* Incidence of hospitalized rhabdomyolysis in patients treated with lipid-lowering drugs. *JAMA* 2004; **292**: 2585–2590.

17. Tanne JH. Meta-analysis says low LDL cholesterol may be associated with greater risk of cancer. *BMJ* 2007; **335**: 177.

18. Poynter JN, Gruber SB, Higging PDR *et al.* Statins and the risk of colorectal cancer. *N Engl J Med* 2005; **352**: 2184–2192.

19. Carlsson CM, Gleason CE, Hess TM *et al.* Effects of simvastatin on cerebrospinal fluid biomarkers and cognition in middle-aged adults at risk for Alzheimer's disease. *J Alzheimers Dis* 2008; **13**: 187–197.

20. Rejnmark L, Vestergaard P, Mosekilde L. Statin but not non-statin lipid-lowering drugs decrease fracture risk: a nation-wide case-control study. *Calcif Tissue Int* 2006; **79**: 29–36.

21. Abramson J, Wright JM. Are lipid-lowering guidelines evidence-based? *Lancet* 2007; **369**: 168–169.

22. McGill Jr HC, McMahan A, Gidding SS. Preventing heart disease in the 21st century: implications of the pathobiological determinants of atherosclerosis in youth (PDAY) study. *Circulation* 2008; **117**: 1216–1227.

23. Frontini MG, Srinivasan SR, Xu JH *et al.* Utility of non-high-density lipoprotein cholesterol versus other lipoprotein measures in detecting subclinical atherosclerosis in young adults (The Bogalusa Heart Study). *Am J Cardiol* 2007; **100**: 64–68.

24. Stein EA, Illingworth DR, Kwiterovich PO *et al.* Efficacy and safety of lovastatin in adolescent males with heterozygous familial hypercholesterolemia. *JAMA* 1999; **281**: 137–144.

25. Green O, Durrington P. Clinical management of children and young adults with heterozygous familial hypercholesterolaemia in the UK. *J R Soc Med* 2004; **97**: 226–229.

26. Knipscheer HC, Boelen CCA, Kastelein JJP *et al.* Short-term efficacy and safety of pravastatin in 72 children with familial hypercholesterolaemia. *Pediatr Res* 1996; **39**: 867–871.

27. Belay B, Belamarich PF, Tom-Revzon C. The use of statins in paediatrics: knowledge base, limitations, and future directions. *Pediatrics* 2007; **119**: 370–380.

28. Neil HA, Huxley RR, Hawkins MM, Durring PN, Betteridge DJ, Humphries SE; Simon Broome Familial Hyperlipidaemia Register Group and Scientific Steering Committee. Comparison of the risk of fatal coronary heart disease in treated xanthomatous and non-xanthomatous heterozygous familial hypercholesterolaemia: a prospective registry study. *Atherosclerosis* 2003; **170**: 73–78.

29. de Jongh S, Lilien MR, op't Roodt J *et al.* Early statin therapy restores endothelial function in children with familial hypercholesterolemia. *J Am Coll Cardiol* 2002; **40**: 2117–2121.

30. Weigman A, Hutten BA, de Groot E *et al.* Efficacy and safety of statin therapy in children with familial hypercholesterolemia: a randomized trial. *JAMA* 2004; **292**: 331–337.

31. Sanjad SA, Al-Abbad A, Al-Shorafa S. Management of hyperlipidemia in children with refractory nephrotic syndrome: the effect of statin therapy. *J Pediatr* 1997; **130**: 470–474.

32. Butani L, Pai MV, Makker SP. Pilot study describing the use of pravastatin in pediatric renal transplant recipients. *Pediatr Transplant* 2003; **7**: 179–184.

33. Penson MG, Fricker FJ, Thompson JR. Safety and efficacy of pravastatin therapy for the prevention of hyperlipidemia in pediatric and adolescent cardiac transplant recipients. *J*

Heart Lung Transplant 2001; **20**: 611–618.

34. Lisik W, Schoenberg L, Lasky RE, Kahan BD. Statins benefit outcomes of renal transplant recipients on a sirolimus-cyclosporine regimen. *Transplant Proc* 2007; **39**: 3086–3092.

35. American Academy of Pediatrics. Cardiovascular risk reduction in high-risk pediatric populations. *Pediatrics* 2007; **119**: 618–621.

36. Edison RJ, Muenke M. Mechanistic and epidemiologic considerations in the evaluation of adverse birth outcomes following gestational exposure to statins. *Am J Med Genet* 2004; **131A**: 287–298.

37. Daniels SR, Greer FR; Committee on Nutrition. Lipid screening and cardiovascular health in childhood. *Pediatrics* 2008; **122**: 198–208.

38. Sanz J, Fayad ZA. Imaging of atherosclerotic cardiovascular disease. *Nature* 2008; **451**: 953–957.

Richard W. Newton

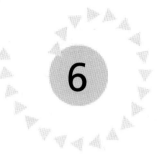

Important advances in Down syndrome

Down syndrome has been recognised for about 150 years, but only recently have we begun to understand its pathogenesis. Research is now accelerating rapidly which should bring benefit for people with and without Down syndrome.

We begin at a school leavers' assembly at a 1500-pupil comprehensive school. Those assembled have a wide range of prospects from aspirant lawyers and teachers, to those with antisocial behaviour orders. One of their number has asked to make a short speech. The 16-year-old begins hesitantly but the 300 gathered listen respectfully. The address is short, clear and poignant, 'I would like to thank everybody for helping me and being my friend'. There is rapturous applause. The boy leaves the stage, a little self-consciously but with a look of satisfaction. The gathering offers genuine warmth and delight in response to the lad's words.

The remarkable thing is that the boy in question has Down syndrome and has just passed through mainstream education. He has known support from his teachers, and peer group. This reflects a sea-change in societal attitude. In 1992, we opened our previous *Recent Advances* chapter on Down syndrome[1] only 11 years after the 1981 Education Act entitled children with a learning disability to an education. 'Mongol' was only just leaving common parlance and a prejudicial view often entered decision-making processes: sub-optimal treatments were reported for heart disease and leukaemia. As you will see, this has all changed, reflecting a view that people with Down syndrome are people with prospects, with a contribution to make who deserve respect, love and support.

Richard W. Newton
Consultant Paediatric Neurologist, Royal Manchester Children's Hospital, Pendlebury, Manchester M27 4HA, UK
E-mail: richard.newton@cmmc.nhs.uk

ADVANCES IN MOLECULAR BIOLOGY

The DNA sequence of about 225 genes on chromosome 21 is now complete. Various mechanisms may contribute to Down syndrome phenotype variability:[2,3] gene expression variability, transcription factor activity (on chromosome 21 or on the genome elsewhere), copy number polymorphisms, the function of conserved non-genomic regions, microRNA activities, RNA editing and, perhaps, DNA methylation. Therapeutic strategies will only result when these effects of gene-dosage imbalance are better understood.

Chromosome 21 is acrocentric with two arms and its centromere close to one end. The short arm 21p consists of the nucleolar organiser region containing multiple gene copies coding for ribosomal RNA and a more proximal region composed of highly repetitive DNA sequences. At least 94 known genes are currently mapped to the long arm (21q). Up to 60% of human genes contribute to the development and/or function of the central nervous system. Thus, between 110 and 150 genes on 21q are probably expressed in the brain and spinal cord (Table 1).

How genes interplay during brain development is yet to be defined. Brain growth often appears normal up to 5–6 months of postnatal life and then decelerates. The result is a foreshortened brain, with reduced frontal lobe volume, occipital flattening and a narrow superior temporal gyrus. Primary cortical gyri appear wide and secondary gyri are poorly developed with a

Table 1 Some chromosome 21 genes expressed in the CNS

Amyloid precursor protein Superoxide dismutase (SOD-1) S100β protein	Functions in signal transduction pathways which regulate the cell cycle and neuronal differentiation
Glutamate receptor sub unit 5	An important excitatory neurotransmitter which mediates dendritic outgrowth and synaptogenesis
Single-minded gene	Codes for a basic helix-loop-helix nuclear protein expressed in the precursor cells of the CNS midline, required for synchronised cell division and the establishment of proper cell lineage
Mini brain gene	Regulates cell cycle kinetics during cell division, expressed during neuroblast proliferation
Systatin B	Expressed in the form of progressive myoclonic epilepsy
GARS-AIRS-GART	Protein complex which catalyses the 2nd, 3rd and 5th steps in *de novo* purine synthesis expressed during cerebellum development (in Down syndrome continues for several postnatal months)
Purkinje cell protein	Expressed in the cerebellum but function unknown
Down syndrome cell adhesion molecule (DSAM)	See below

small cerebellum and brain stem. Neuronal proliferation, differentiation and organisation are all affected but myelination only variably. Hypocellularity is due to a reduction in neurone proliferation and increased neuronal apoptosis.[3] Increased glutathione peroxidase and superoxide dismutase-1 (SOD-1) activity is associated with increased lipid peroxidation. Fetal Down syndrome neurones exhibit a 3–4-fold increase in reactive oxygen species and elevated levels of lipid peroxidation *in vitro* before the onset of degeneration and cell death, occurring as early as 25 weeks' gestation. The effects of chronically increased membrane lipid peroxidation on synaptic and cellular function may be particularly important in understanding how neurocognitive decline occurs in adult life in association with the neuropathological features of Alzheimer's disease.[3]

BRAIN DEVELOPMENT: NEURONAL MIGRATION

Genes govern the migration of 100,000 million neurones from the rostral end of the embryonic neural tube. Growth cones[4] appear at the axonal tips, and wriggle their dynamic cytoskeleton, an exoskeleton of cell-movement molecules, notably actin. They are directed by extracellular information including mechanical forces, their response to neurotransmitters and other three-dimensional biochemical gradients, conditioned by specific genes expressing themselves at a particular phase of neuronal development. In addition to this matrix constituent responsiveness (the local micro-environment encountered at any one particular time), the neurones make contact with the membranes of other cells and axons. In this process, they are supported by a set of cell adhesion molecules. The Down syndrome cell adhesion molecule is one of the most studied.[2,3]

The gene coding the Down syndrome cell adhesion molecule (DSAM) comprises 24 exons.[4] Mutually exclusive alternative splicing may occur for exons 4, 6, 9 and 17. One of 12 exon 4 alternatives, one of 48 exon 6 alternatives, one of 33 exon 9 alternatives and one of 2 exon 17 alternatives are retained in each mRNA. You can perm any four from 60: this leads to a massive number of potential Down syndrome cell adhesion molecules. This means growth cones are very specific for their ultimate target.

Many other molecules are involved in intercellular signalling and axon guidance; the semiphorins (clearly named by a former scout!), ephrins and their Eph receptors, slit proteins along with gradients for neurotransmitters including γ-aminobutyric acid and glutamate.

It is clear to see how genetic variability in Down syndrome may lead to abnormal targeting, a detrimental effect on neuronal circuitry and a brain with reduced capacity for efficient learning and functioning.

Knowledge of this process allows us to offer parents simple biological explanations for their child's learning disability and not just in Down syndrome. Too often, doctors tell parents 'We just do not know' (what the cause of their child's learning disability is). This leaves many parents dissatisfied and spurs them on to seek further opinions in a quest for some sort of answer. With no magnetic resonance imaging features of brain injury nor any neurometabolic marker (true for at least 6 out of 10 children we see when asked to investigate learning disability), the answer must be that neuronal circuitry fell short of full development due to genetic malfunction at a critical stage in brain development. We can explain to parents how 100,000 million nerve cells have to get from one place to another; how genes tell them when to grow, where to grow and what to join up with. We can illustrate this with simple diagrams. We can mention that in the centre of each nerve cell there are roughly 30,000 genes, any of which has a potential for malfunction. Most parents will then understand how the interplay of a gene or small group of genes might go wrong and how difficult that is to trace. Empirical recurrence risk can still be offered by the clinical geneticists. In this way, the knowledge of a complex process, a significant part of which has been derived from our study of Down syndrome, allows us to help many families.

ANTENATAL SCREENING

Antenatal screening is designed to give women a compound risk factor for an affected baby. Information is integrated from epidemiological factors such as maternal age, pregnancy-specific variables such as serum markers, and fetal-specific variables such as nuchal translucency. These serum markers carry gestational age-specific sensitivities and specificities to predict Down syndrome.[5,6] Statistical modelling allows us to identify which are most efficient and cost-effective at any gestational age, bearing in mind practicalities and individual choice.

All screening should be accompanied by adequate information and counselling so that families can understand the procedures and choices available to them. Currently, free β-human chorionic gonadatrophin (hCG) and pregnancy-associated plasma protein A (PAPP-A) are assayed at 10–14 weeks' gestation in association with ultrasound screening of nuchal translucency. In the second trimester, α-fetoprotein and β-hCG are assayed at 15–20 weeks' gestation though some units also combine unconjugated oestriol (uE3) and inhibin A.[7] When a high risk of abnormality is identified, chorionic villus sampling in the first trimester or amniocentesis beyond 15 weeks' gestation follows. Meanwhile, nasal bone assessment by ultrasound is being evaluated.[8]

GIVING THE NEWS

Giving the news to a family of Down syndrome, a life-threatening or chronic disabling condition is never easy. The principles of how best to carry this out (see Table 2) are now part of the curriculum in most medical schools, a change since 1992, though this will beat neither professional nor life experience.

LANGUAGE TO USE AND AVOID

Chesterton said: 'I do not know what I think about a thing until I hear what I say'. Jokes we tell or phrases we use will too often reflect attitudes held, albeit subconsciously. Careful thought should be given to the words we use in consultations.

'I need to give you some news that none of us was expecting when Jimmy was born' is better than, 'I am really sorry to have to tell you…'. It is better to

Table 2 Giving the news of serious conditions

1. News to be given by a senior and experienced member of the team who, insofar as is possible, knows the family well.

2. Both parents to be present or at least one parent accompanied by another close family member or friend. If not immediately possible, contrive to put the meeting back.

3. The meeting should be held in a private, quiet and uninterrupted setting for which the doctor has cleared sufficient time from the busy schedule to do the job well.

4. The baby should, in so far as is possible, be present to give the message that the baby is valued and part of that family.

5. Simple truthful and factual information should be offered. It should be remembered that most diagnoses are never more than a probability statement with quite a broad attendant spectrum of possible outcome. Remember most parents are feeling acutely anxious once that initial diagnosis is given and may not be receptive to much information at that point. This emphasises the value of forging a new meeting with them in 24 h or so. Written information including the Down Syndrome Association <www.downs-syndrome.org.uk> is very useful at this stage. If the midwife, health visitor or social worker known to the family is also present he or she can help parents recount some of the information given and formulate questions that might be asked at that next meeting, or indeed subsequently.

use neutral and non-judgmental phrases. Address your own fears and prejudices. The vast majority of families find a way forward and continue to thrive with everyone ultimately learning to laugh again. You would probably be the same. Try to convey that confidence to the families involved. Refer to 'children with Down syndrome', rather than 'Down syndrome children' (there is the world of difference!).

Do not infer that remedial therapy will put anything right but is rather about creating opportunity and avoiding secondary disadvantage. A child with Down syndrome is no different from any other: to reach their potential, they need love, opportunity and encouragement – nature will do the rest. Tell parents to have confidence in themselves as the child's teacher. Other family members, friends and professionals will all give advice. Teach them to have the confidence to choose what is right for them.

Most parents go through a bereavement reaction of some sort. They shed tears for the child they were expecting rather than the one who actually arrived. Help them recognise these feelings as being quite separate from their new baby (who they will get to know and love). Mothers and fathers may work through their grief at different rates. Help them recognise this and remind them they have to be nice to each other! Assure them that they will grow strong and the family will learn to laugh again. The family may well develop a degree of psychological dependence on any person giving this sort of advice for a while. Try to be available and responsive to that occasional phone call.

Now let us consider how some scientific advances might be applied to clinical practice.

CONGENITAL HEART DISEASE

THE GENETIC APPROACH

Significant progress has been made in our understanding of the molecular and genetic determinants of congenital heart defects (CHDs).[9] CHD is seen in 40–50% of people with Down syndrome and anatomical patterns are specific. For example, a complete atrioventricular canal defect affects about 75% of those with a heart defect but without left-sided obstructive lesions seen more commonly in those without Down syndrome. Ventriculoseptal defects are common but usually perimembranous whereas muscular and sub-arterial septal defects are rare. Tetralogy of Fallot may be found in 10–15%. Interestingly, some CHDs such as L-loop of the ventricles, atresia of the atrioventricular valves and transposition of the great arteries are virtually absent in Down syndrome, suggesting that genetic variants may be protective.

As with the brain, cell adhesion plays an important role in heart morphogenesis. Fetal trisomy 21 hearts show more intense staining of type VI collagen than normal hearts suggesting a potential mechanism for developmental defect. Compelling candidates for atrioventricular canal defects (AVSDs) on chromosome 21 are the *Col 6A1* and *Col 6A2* gene clusters which, respectively, encode the alpha-1 and alpha-2 chains for type VI collagen.[10] Other studies have shown that the primary anatomical basis of the AVSDs is often reduced expansion of the vestibular spine derived from the dorsal mesocardium with perhaps secondary or at times a primary failure of fusion of the endocardial cushions. Understanding the different developmental courses that can lead to AVSDs will be of value in the search for genes that increase susceptibility to this condition.

With new genetic knowledge some new terms are emerging. 'Reversal medicine' refers to how new sensitive and specific diagnostic genetic criteria may, in the future, prove to be more useful than anatomical and clinical criteria used for phenotyping hitherto. The anatomical genetic classification of the AVCDs in Down syndrome is one example. 'Predictive medicine' relates prognosis to genotype, for example, genetic syndromes and surgical outcome. In children with tetralogy of Fallot, Down syndrome is not a risk factor for outcome of surgery. This approach allows specific peri-operative protocols to be applied to reduce risk and more accurate counselling to be provided in prenatal life.

An example of 'predictive medicine' is seen in the study of 106 consecutive repairs of a complete artrioventriculoseptal defect.[11] The overall mortality was 7.7% (6% among those with Down syndrome and 14% among those without Down syndrome). The only independent risk factor affecting survival was the presence of unbalanced ventricles; a Norwood procedure (a series of three operations designed to correct under-development of left heart tissue by using grafts alongside right heart tissue) was more frequently needed amongst those with Down syndrome as was the prevalence of pulmonary artery banding. Re-operation was required much less frequently in those without Down syndrome due to a lesser incidence of mitral valve anomaly. The study indicates that with the improved care process Down syndrome no longer increases the risk of biventricular repair.

UPPER AIRWAY DISEASE

A number of Down syndrome features predispose to obstructive sleep apnoea syndrome and otitis media. These include infection susceptibility, adenotonsilar hypertrophy, macroglosia, mid-facial hypoplasia, muscular hypotension and, in a few, hypothyroidism and obesity.

More research is required to define how best to treat middle-ear infection and deafness in children with Down syndrome. Recent Cochrane reviews assessing antibiotic therapy and antihistamines[12,13] showed neither to be better than placebo in shortening the illness or reducing longer term complications. Paediatricians should be aware that middle-ear deafness is prevalent in Down syndrome, and that regular testing is required to minimise the impact, as language disorder is common.

Marcus and colleagues[14] studied 53 children with Down syndrome and found that 60% had sleep-related upper airway obstruction. The commonest abnormality was hypoventilation with 80% showing an elevated carbon dioxide level during an overnight polysomnogram. An Oxfordshire study[15] of 32 children with Down syndrome showed about a third had at least three symptoms suggestive of sleep-related problems, the commonest being snoring and chest wall recession. In addition, 41% had a pattern of increased inspiratory resistance compared to 3% of controls. Two-thirds had oxygen saturation levels below those of controls. In its extreme form, children may present with pulmonary hypertension or even right heart failure though this may be preceded by less-specific features including swallowing difficulties, recurrent upper respiratory tract infections, nausea and vomiting, day-time sleepiness, persistent or secondary enuresis, nocturnal sweating, cyanosis or apnoea. If suspicions arise, polysomnography is the gold standard investigation usually requiring referral to a specialist unit. Ahead of that, a video tape to observe the child's behaviour during sleep, pulse oximetry, inspiratory resistance and carbon dioxide measurements may all add useful information.

Watchful waiting with topical decongestants or steroid is often a suitable initial approach. Following this, due consideration ought to be given to adenotonsilectomy and than nasal CPAP (not always well tolerated in this group!).[16]

LOWER RESPIRATORY TRACT DISEASE

A community-based Australian study identified 8% of children with Down syndrome to have significant lower respiratory illness.[17] The majority of children with Down syndrome required hospital admission before their 16th birthday and a respiratory problem was the cause for admission in over half; congenital heart disease was present in only a third and 1 in 10 required intensive care.[18] Hypotonia, obesity, cardiac disease and immune dysfunction may all contribute. Congenital anomalies of the lower airways are also common (strongly associated with cardiovascular anomalies) which may be stenotic or malacic (airway collapse) anomalies, tracheo-oesophageal fistula or branching anomalies.[19] Gastro-oesophageal reflux disease needs to be excluded.

Tracheal and pulmonary hypoplasia and/or sub-pleural cysts are all more common in Down syndrome than in the general population. Consider significant lower respiratory tract disease with a history of recurrent infections, wheeze, stridor (with or without cough), failure to extubate, sudden collapse, disproportionate ventilatory requirement or corticosteroid/β-agonist resistant lung disease.

Investigations should include a good assessment of cardiac status, the patency of the upper airway, complete blood count and immunoglobulins, upper gastrointestinal contrast studies with a 24-h pH probe to rule out significant gastro-oesophageal reflux disease proceeding as necessary to flexible bronchoscopy and imaging (usually computed tomography) of the lungs. The mainstays of management are to treat significant reflux aggressively, continuous prophylactic antibiotics and regular inhaled glucocorticoids. This should be complemented by physiotherapy and non-invasive ventilation (in selected cases), as appropriate.[19]

ENDOCRINE DISORDERS

DIABETES

Type 1 diabetes is around 10 times more common in children with Down syndrome than in the general population. It often develops early with around 20% presenting before the age of 2 years. The presentation is acute and often difficult to manage but the approach to management is as for other children. The genetic mechanism is not clear but autoimmunity probably plays an important part (see below).

A diabetes susceptibility study in Down syndrome may allow a greater understanding of the disorder in the general population. Gillespie and colleagues[20] showed the frequency of sub-clinical islet autoimmunity is increased in Down syndrome and susceptibility to type I diabetes partially HLA-mediated through an excess of diabetes-associated HLA class II genotypes compared with age- and sex-matched healthy control subjects in the general population. Children with Down syndrome and type I diabetes were, however, less likely to carry the highest risk genotype DR4-DQ8/DRD3-DQ2. Other genetic factors may increase the penetrance of type I diabetes in Down syndrome.

THYROID DISEASE

Congenital hypothyroidism

There is an unexplained higher incidence of congenital hypothyroidism in Down syndrome. The mean T4 concentration in children with Down syndrome is normally distributed but shifted to lower concentrations, unexplained by prematurity, non-thyroid illness or iodine exposure. Mean thyroid stimulating hormone and T4 binding globulin concentrations are significantly increased and normal, respectively. This all points to a mild hypothyroid state in Down syndrome newborns suggesting a Down syndrome-specific thyroid regulation disorder.[21] However, a double-blind, controlled trial investigating the effects of thyroid treatment on development and growth of young children with Down syndrome identified no benefit for cognitive development and a small, but rather unimportant, gain for motor development (0.7 months in 2 years) at age 24 months.[22] Thyroxine-treated children had greater gains in length and weight (1.1 cm at 378 g in 2 years).

Isolated raised thyroid stimulating hormone

About 30% of people with Down syndrome will develop some aspect of thyroid function test abnormality under the age of 22 years. This has led many to advocate annual screening for thyroid disease or treatment where raised thyroid stimulating hormone levels are found in the face of a normal T4. The reason for this is not clear; thyroid stimulating hormone bioactivity is exactly the same in Down syndrome as it is in the general population.[23] Gibson and colleagues[24] followed a cohort of 122 children with Down syndrome through the first two decades. At first testing, 24 had isolated raised thyroid stimulating hormone levels; 20 were retested and 14 (70%) had become normal. Seventeen with isolated raised thyroid stimulating hormone levels on initial testing had a thyrotrophin releasing hormone test within 3 months; the thyroid stimulating hormone level had become normal in 8 (47%) of these children. There was no association between reported clinical symptoms and isolated raised thyroid stimulating hormone level but there were clear symptoms in one of the two with definite hypothyroidism. It was noted that the likelihood ratio for a positive result on second testing when raised thyroid stimulating hormone level and positive antibody status on first testing are combined is 20. This suggests initial testing results could be used as a basis to select a subgroup for further testing at say 5-yearly intervals unless new symptoms emerge in the interim. The results also suggest that annual screening (as recommended by the American Academy of Pediatrics in 2001) are probably not justified in the first 20 years of life. Certainly, isolated raised thyroid stimulating hormone appears not to be a risk factor for cardiac disease,[25] indicating intervention cannot be justified on this score.

HAEMATOLOGICAL DISORDERS

TRANSIENT ABNORMAL MYELOPOIESIS

Transient abnormal myelopoiesis is virtually unique to Down syndrome[26] and presents in fetal (anaemia causing heart failure and hydrops-fetalis) or neonatal life. In neonatal life, transient abnormal myelopoiesis usually presents with circulating blast cells with or without a mild leukocytosis. The indication for blood tests is usually bruising, skin infiltrates, pleural, pericardial or peritoneal effusions, respiratory distress or hepatomegaly which may be associated with jaundice. The haemoglobin is often normal but thrombocytopenia is common, the characteristic blood film feature being deeply basophilic immature blast cells (rather like those seen in premature babies but in much greater numbers).

Most children with transient abnormal myelopoiesis simply require watchful waiting. However, symptomatic babies may require treatment with low-dose cytosine-arabinoside. Severe liver disease with fibrosis has a poor prognosis and the mortality may be up to 20%. Some 20–30% will proceed to develop myeloid leukaemia of Down syndrome. Neonates with transient abnormal myelopoiesis have mutations in the key megakaryocyte transcription factor GATA1. In the majority, there is spontaneous resolution. Prospective studies are required to identify its true incidence and associated morbidity and mortality.

MYELOID LEUKAEMIA OF DOWN SYNDROME

This presents between 1–4 years of age and most have preceding transient abnormal myelopoiesis.[26] The child usually becomes progressively anaemic and thrombocytopenic with dysplastic changes in the erythroid cell and megakaryocytes. Historically, there was a very poor prognosis but now a favourable response to low doses of cytarabine has been recognised. Five-year survival rates of 80% are recorded. Treatment failure is usually due to mucositis or infection.

ACUTE LYMPHOBLASTIC LEUKAEMIA OF DOWN SYNDROME

This is much more common in children than acute myeloid leukaemia[26] and clinical features of acute lymphoblastic leukaemia are similar in children with or without Down syndrome. Therefore, more than 90% have a precursor B-cell immunophenotype and T-cell disease is relative uncommon. However, in Down syndrome, acute lymphoblastic leukaemia is more likely to have adverse (hypodiplody) rather than favourable prognostic karyotype (hyperdiplody and t(12.21)). Outcome is not as good as in children without Down syndrome (60–70% cured as opposed to 75–85%). This has lead to more aggressive treatment but, unfortunately, greater toxicities are encountered. In contrast to myeloid leukaemia of Down syndrome, there is no evidence of increased sensitivity of the leukaemia to the treatments and mucositis and infection are the common determinants of death.[26]

SKELETAL ABNORMALITIES

The hypotonia of Down syndrome linked to a degree of ligamentous laxity leads to mobile and, at times, aching joints. Regular exercise prevents muscle atrophy and promotes joint stability. The common posture in the lower limb is that of pes planus with valgus at the ankle. A medial arch support tends to throw weight on to the outer arch and to correct the valgus at the ankle. This leads to a better base for movement, greater stability and fewer aching feet. Analgesia can be used sensibly.

The tendency to atlanto-axial instability with the attendant risk of dislocation demands special consideration. In 1995, the American Academy of Pediatrics indicated atlanto-axial instability met no accepted criteria for a screening programme to be worthwhile, thus modifying its earlier stance. The condition is extremely rare (41 cases reported by 1995, world-wide), offering little justification for the resources required for its detection in the asymptomatic phase. The screening test should have good sensitivity and specificity for asymptomatic atlanto-axial instability, which in turn should be a proven risk factor for symptomatic atlanto-axial instability.[27] Reproducibility of the radiological screening test is poor[28] unless great attention is given to conditions in which the X-rays are taken.[29] When 90 children aged 4–19 years were followed for 5 years there was an significant reduction in the atlanto-axial gap. However, the one child who developed acute symptomatic atlanto-axial instability after ear, nose and throat surgery had had a previously normal cervical spine X-ray. Despite all of this, in 2007 the Special Olympics Committee still requires a temporary restriction of individuals with Down syndrome from participation in activities that 'pose potential risk' including butterfly stroke and diving starts in swimming, soccer, high jump and skiing unless an X-ray has excluded atlanto-axial instability or two physicians certify that participation is appropriate.

The author believes that screening in this way is inappropriate and offers an infringement of personal liberty. The one thing that does need emphasising, however, is the potential risk for all people with Down syndrome under anaesthesia. It is essential that all anaesthetists are aware of the potential risk of extending the neck no matter what procedure is being undertaken.

IMMUNE DISORDERS

In children with Down syndrome the activation, proliferation and maturation of T- and B-lymphocytes in response to encounters with environmental antigens is severely diminished.[30] T-lymphocyte sub-population counts gradually rise reaching more mature levels in time, but the B-lymphocyte population remains severely diminished with 88% of values falling below the 10th centile and 61% below the 5th centile. Thymic alterations are described in Down syndrome that could explain decreased T-lymphocyte numbers but not the striking B-lymphocytopenia. Both lymphocyte function-associated antigen-1 and intracellular adhesion molecule-1 are over-expressed in the thymus in Down syndrome, but the exact role of these molecules in determining the size of T-cell populations is unknown though increased immature lymphocyte deletion is a possibility.[31] It is also reported that the specific loss of Down syndrome cell adhesion molecule impairs the efficiency of bacterial uptake by phagocytes. Studies of Down syndrome cell adhesion molecule, SOD-1 gene over-expression, T-cell deficiency, decreased B-cell maturation, an increased susceptibility to bacterial and viral infections performed over the past decade provide support for the hypothesis that chromosome gene over-expression leads to the impaired interaction between immature thymocytes and thymic strobal cells.[32]

Children with Down syndrome and sepsis have an elevated mortality rate of 1.333, after confounding factors such as demographics, pathogens and co-morbidity are controlled. The Oxford Record Linkage Study[34] concluded that the risk for cancers combined (excluding leukaemia) was not significantly elevated (1.2; 0.6 to 2.2); the risk of testicular cancer was increased (12; 2.5 to 35.6) – but a risk based on only three subjects whilst Patja and colleagues[35] observed low incidence of solid tumours in individuals with Down syndrome. However, significantly elevated risks were found for celiac disease (4.7; 1.3 to 12.2), acquired hypothyroidism (9.4; 3.4 to 20.5), other thyroid disorders and type I diabetes mellitus (2.8; 1 to 6.1). Interestingly, a decreased risk for asthma was observed (0.4; 0.2 to 0.6).[34] Clearly, further study of basic immunology and epidemiology in Down syndrome is required to help understand the mechanisms responsible for these important associations, in particular to delineate the relative contributions of premature ageing (see below) and inherent immune defect.

AUTOIMMUNITY

About 40% of children with Down syndrome have thyroid autoantibodies aged 1–20 years (30% developing abnormalities of thyroid function including isolated raised thyroid stimulating hormone). Whereas HLA locus is not associated with thyroid disease in the general population, it does appear to be in those with Down syndrome indicating some sort of permissive effect of chromosome 21.[36]

IgA-positive antibodies (antigliadin antibodies) are present in about a quarter of those with Down syndrome compared to about 1% of the general population; with 1 in 3 of the antigliadin antibody positive children having total villus atrophy.[37] This means that 5–12%[37,38] of young people with Down syndrome have celiac disease. Autoimmunity in type I diabetes in Down syndrome has already been discussed.

A number of genes mapped to chromosome 21 might confer autoimmunity. AIRE (auto-immune regulator) causes autoimmune polyglandular syndrome type 1. It is known that disomic homozygosity does not occur but over expression may, nonetheless, be important. Amyloid precursor protein in association with SOD-1 over-expression is associated with β-amyloid deposition, increased cell death due to apoptosis and, probably, increased reactive oxygen free radicals. Increased tissue destruction and associated inflammation may increase the risk of organ damage with lymphocytic infiltration. Although superoxide levels are reduced within the tissues, the result is an increase in hydroxal ions which can be as damaging. Ligand of ICOS is part of a co-stimulatory mechanism which facilitates antigen-presenting cells interacting with T-cells. The result is proliferation and cytokine reduction and, therefore, more tissue damage and inflammation (on CD4[+] and CD8[+] cells).

VITAMIN THERAPY

Many parents feel a strong compulsion to 'do something to put the Down syndrome right'. Thankfully, the days when parents would opt for 'Sicca cell therapy' (an injection of dried fetal embryo cells) or plastic surgery (to 'make them look more normal') seems now to have passed. There are also advocates of vitamin therapy, despite the fact that Down syndrome is associated with gene over-expression and co-enzymes might be harmful. A recent systematic review[39] of 11 trials involving 373 randomised participants studied the effect of dietary supplementation and/or drugs with improved cognitive function as the outcome measure. The quality of the trials was poor but none of the comparisons showed a cognitive enhancing effect. On theoretical grounds, antioxidants might be beneficial (vitamin E or zinc to enhance glucothione reductase activity) but the effect is only likely to be seen very long term. This makes good study design difficult. The most likely source of direction in this respect is animal studies with consensus statements but current knowledge does not allow us to recommend any particular antioxidant in any particular dosage.

Key points for clinical practice

- Screening programmes should incorporate counselling, information, practicality and individual choice.

- When giving diagnostic news, mind your language.

- Therapeutic strategies will only result when the effects of gene dosage imbalance are better understood.

- Predictive medicine allows surveillance in the most vulnerable.

- Reversal medicine refers to how genetic criteria may prove more useful than anatomical and clinical criteria for phenotyping.

- The study of subjects with Down syndrome may well lead to a better understanding of disease in the general population. This certainly applies to morphogenesis of heart lesions, immune disorders and autoimmunity in particularly.

- Sleep-related upper airway obstruction and lower respiratory disease is common in Down syndrome.

- If a child with Down syndrome has symptoms, investigate and treat them as you would any child.

- Anaesthesia in Down syndrome is high risk: remind the anaesthetist.

- Think of celiac disease as one cause of failure to thrive in Down syndrome.

- Transient abnormal myelopoiesis is almost certainly a pre-leukaemic condition related to myeloid leukaemia of Down syndrome and associated with GATA1 mutations.

- Diabetes is 10 times more common in Down syndrome than in the general population and presents early.

References

1: Newton RW, Newton JA. Management of Down's syndrome. In: David TF. (ed) *Recent Advances in Paediatrics*. Edinburgh: Churchill Livingstone, 1992; 21–35.
2. Patterson D. Genetic mechanisms involved in the phenotype of Down syndrome. *Mental Retard Dev Disabil Res Rev* 2007; **13**: 199–206.
3. Capone GT. Down syndrome: advances in molecular biology and the neurosciences. *Dev Behav Pediatr* 2001; **22**: 40–59.
4. Schmucker D, Clemens JC, Shu H *et al*. *Drosophila* Dscam is an axon guidance receptor exhibiting extraordinary molecular diversity. *Cell* 2000; **101**: 671–684.
5. Cuckle H. Integrating antenatal Down's syndrome screening. *Curr Opin Obstet Gynecol* 2001; **13**: 175–181.

6. Sheppard C, Platt LD. Nuchal translucency and first trimester risk assessment. A systematic review. *Ultrasound Q* 2007; **23**: 107–116.
7. <http://www.fetalanomaly.screening.nhs.uk/screening>.
8. Rosen T, D'Alton ME, Platt LD, Wapner R. First-trimester ultrasound assessment of the nasal bone to screen for aneuploidy. *Obstet Gynecol* 2007; **110**: 399–404.
9. Piacentinia GM, Digiliob C, Sarkozyc A, Placidia S, Dallapiccolac B, Marinoa B. Genetics of congenital heart diseases in syndromic and non-syndromic patients: new advances and clinical implications. *J Cardiovasc Med* 2007; **8**: 7–11.
10. Maslen CM. Molecular genetics of atrioventricular septal defects. *Curr Opin Cardiol* 2004; **19**: 205–210.
11. Formigari R, Di Donato RM, Gargiulo G *et al*. Better surgical prognosis for patients with complete atrioventricular septal defect and Down's syndrome. *Ann Thorac Surg* 2004; **78**: 666–672.
12. Glasziou PP, Del Mar CB, Sanders SL, Hayem M. Antibiotics for acute otitis media in children. Cochrane Database Syst Rev 1997, Issue 1. CD000219.
13. Griffin GH, Flynn C, Bailey RE, Schultz JK. Antihistamines and/or decongestants for otitis media with effusion (OME) in children. Cochrane Database Syst Rev 2006, Issue 4. CD003423.
14. Marcus CL, Keens TG, Bautista DB, von Pechmann WS, Ward SL. Obstructive sleep apnea in children with Down syndrome. *Pediatrics* 1991; **88**: 132–139.
15. Stebbens VA, Dennis J, Samuels MP, Croft CB, Southall DP. Sleep related upper airway obstruction in a cohort with Down's syndrome. *Arch Dis Child* 1991; **66**: 1333–1338.
16. Samuels M. Sleep related upper airways obstruction in Down's syndrome: diagnostic approaches and treatment. 2001. Conference proceedings. <http://www.dsmig.org.uk/library/articles/transcript-samuels.pdf>.
17. Selikowitz M. Health problems and health checks in school-aged children with Down's syndrome. *J Paediatr Child Health* 1992; **28**: 383–386.
18. Hilton JM, Fitzgerald DA, Cooper DM. Respiratory morbidity of hospitalised children with trisomy 21. *J Paediatr Child Health* 1999; **35**: 383–386.
19. Doull I. Respiratory disorders in Down's syndrome: overview with diagnostic and treatment options. Conference proceedings 2001. <http://www.dsmig.org.uk/library/articles/transcript-doull.pdf>.
20. Gillespie KM, Dix RJ, Williams AJK *et al*. Islet autoimmunity in children with Down's syndrome. *Diabetes* 2006; **55**: 3185–3188.
21. van Trotsenburg ASP, Vulsma T, van Santen HM, Cheung W, de Vijlder JJM. Lower neonatal screening thyroxine concentrations in Down syndrome newborns. *J Clin Endocrinol Metab* 2003; **88**: 1512–1515.
22. van Trotsenburg ASP, Vulsma T, Rutgers van Rozenburg-Marres SL *et al*. The effect of thyroxine treatment started in the neonatal period on development and growth of two-year-old Down syndrome children: a randomized clinical trial. *J Clin Endocrinol Metab* 2005; **90**: 3304–3311.
23. Konings CH, van Trotsenburg AS, Ris-Staplers C, Vulsma T, Wiedijk BM, de Vijlder JJ. Plasma thyrotropin bioactivity in Down's syndrome children with subclinical hypothyroidism. *Eur J Endocrinol* 2001; **144**: 1–4.
24. Gibson PA, Newton RW, Selby K, Price DA, Leyland K, Addison GM. Longitudinal study of thyroid function in Down's syndrome in the first two decades. *Arch Dis Child* 2005; **90**: 574–578.
25. Toscano E, Pacileo G, Limongelli G *et al*. Subclinical hypothyroidism and Down's syndrome; studies on myocardial structure and function. *Arch Dis Child* 2003; **88**: 1005–1008.
26. Webb D, Roberts I, Vyas P. Haematology of Down syndrome. *Arch Dis Child* 2007; **92**: F503–F507.
27. Committee on Sports Medicine and Fitness of the American Academy of Pediatrics. Atlanto-axial instability in Down syndrome: subject review. *Pediatrics* 1995; **96**: 151–154.
28. Selby SM, Newton RW, Gupta S, Hunt L. Clinical predictors and radiologic reliability in atlanto-axial subluxation in Down's syndrome. *Arch Dis Child* 1991; **66**: 876–878.
29. Morton RE, Khan MA, Marie-Leslie C, Elliott S. Atlanto-axial instability in Down syndrome: a five year follow up study. *Arch Dis Child* 1995; **72**: 115–118.

30. de Hingh YCM, van der Vossen PW, Gemen EFA *et al*. Intrinsic abnormalities of lymphocyte counts in children with Down syndrome. *J Pediatr* 2005; **147**: 744–747.
31. Douglas SD. Down syndrome: immunologic and epidemiologic associations – enigmas remain. *J Pediatr* 2005; **147**: 723–725.
32. Murphy M, Insoft RM, Pike-Nobile L, Epstein LB. A hypothesis to explain the immune defects in Down syndrome. *Prog Clin Biol Res* 1995; **393**: 147–167.
33. Garrison MM, Jeffries H, Christakis DA. Risk of death for children with and without Down syndrome who have sepsis. *J Pediatr* 2005; **147**: 748–752.
34. Goldacre MJ, Wotton CJ, Seagroatt V, Yeates D. Cancers and immune related diseases associated with Down syndrome: a record linkage study. *Arch Dis Child* 2004; **89**: 1014–1017.
35. Patja K, Pukkala E, Sund R *et al*. Cancer incidence of persons with Down syndrome in Finland: a population-based study. *Int J Cancer* 2006; **118**: 1769–1772.
36. Nicholson LB, Wong FS, Ewins DL *et al*. Susceptibility to autoimmune thyroiditis in Down's syndrome is associated with the major histocompatibility class II DQA 0301 allele. *Clin Endocrinol* 1994; **41**: 381–383.
37. Castro M, Crino A, Papadatou B *et al*. Down's syndrome and celiac disease: the prevalence of high IgA-antigliadin antibodies and HLA-DR and DQ antigens in trisomy 21. *J Pediatr Gastroenterol Nutr* 1993; **16**: 265–268.
38. Failla P, Ruberto C, Pagano MC *et al*. Celiac disease in Down's syndrome with HLA serological and molecular studies. *J Pediatr Gastroenterol Nutr* 1996; **23**: 303–306.
39. Salman MS. Systematic review of the effect of therapeutic dietary supplements and drugs on cognitive function in subjects with Down syndrome. *Eur J Paediatr Neurol* 2002; **6**: 213–219.

Jacob Levitt

7

Head lice

The diagnosis of head lice is all too often dismissed by the physician as a nuisance (while simultaneously eliciting revulsion and a hope that the patient stays as far away as possible from the office). It is equally and oppositely exaggerated by the patient, who exhibits disgust, embarrassment, and a desire to purge all things close to them of anything creepy-crawly. That said, to appreciate the patient perspective, please imagine yourself with head lice – six-legged insects, crawling and defecating digested blood in your hair, biting your scalp, potentially infesting your child and your spouse, and going with you to every place you hold private and singularly your space – your favourite coat and hat, your office, your bed.

The extreme emotion generated by the diagnosis of head lice, coupled with a lack of knowledge by all parties involved, leads to the propagation of various myths concerning head lice. Ignorance leads to exaggerated perceptions of their transmissibility, elevating useless and potentially dangerous products to the status of efficacious, and deeming efficacious ones as so extremely hurtful as to be unfit for human use.

This chapter will attempt to provide an evidence-based approach to the diagnosis and treatment of lice. From an understanding of the head lice life cycle, mechanism of action of the various treatment alternatives, and current resistance profiles of head lice flows a rational strategy for the management of head lice infestations.

IMPORTANCE OF THERAPY

Reasons to treat head lice are manifold: (i) louse-associated pruritus and rash; (ii) psychosocial and economic impact to patient and family; and (iii)

Jacob Levitt MD
Assistant Clinical Professor, Department of Dermatology, The Mount Sinai Medical Center, 5 East 98th Street, Fifth Floor, Box 1048, New York, NY 10029, USA
E-mail: jacob.levitt@mountsinai.org

prevention of bacterial scalp pyoderma and theoretical prevention of blood born viral and bacterial pathogens.

LOUSE-ASSOCIATED PRURITUS AND RASH

Itching is the primary manifestation of head louse infestation. In severe infestations, a patient might lose sleep due to pruritus. A child may not report itching *per se* but can be seen repeatedly scratching his or her head. Arthropod bite reactions, manifested as red papules, sometimes occur. These are typically found in the posterior scalp and neck and behind the ears. While never formally proven, the red papules are felt to be due to an immune response to the louse saliva.[1] Rarely, papular urticaria can occur.

Psychosocial and economic impact to patient and family

Psychosocial pressures of having lice generally mandate effective treatment. Children become self-conscious,[2] parents become anxious and obsessive about the possibility of infestation recurrence, and social contacts are generally disgusted and fearful of continued contact during an infestation.

Given the stigma of head lice, school policy often mandates exclusion of children from school when diagnosed with head lice and until free of infestation. Such policies are hurtful to the child and have little rational basis from a medical standpoint. The criteria for diagnosis vary from school to school. Some define it specifically (visualising live lice), while others define it broadly – the presence of nits (whether viable or non-viable).

Because hair grows at 1 cm/month,[3] and because most lice need to lay eggs close to the scalp where it is relatively warm and moist, if a nurse detects a nit 2 cm from the scalp, the infestation likely has been there for at least 2 months. Nits alone should not be a factor in school attendance policy since only 18% of school children found to have nits will eventually be diagnosed with an infestation.[4] To banish a child from school the day the infestation is detected is extreme, as the other children have been exposed for 2 months. A more reasonable approach would be to mandate proof of treatment within a week's time.

If you speak to enough school nurses, you will encounter situations where children have been left back an entire year due to head lice-related exclusion from school. While no exact data exist, in the US, one can estimate that 6–24 million days of school were missed due to head lice (assuming 1–2 days of school missed per case and 6–12 million cases per year).[5] When a child misses school, parents must often miss work and/or pay for child care. Schools can lose government money that is contingent upon attendance rates.

Costs of lice therapy include physician visits and therapy. Prescription therapy is felt to be most reliable, albeit more expensive, if payment is out-of-pocket. One should be wary of 'pocket book friendly' folk remedies (mayonnaise, kerosene, *etc.*) and those that prey on patient anxiety (*i.e.*, many professional nit picking services). Less expensive modalities, such as nit combing by varying systems, have variable efficacy. Shaving the head can be emotionally traumatic, but it does work well.[5]

Prevention of lice-associated pathogens

In tropical climates, head lice infestation is the most common cause of scalp pyoderma.[1] In arid climates of developed countries, scalp pyoderma is less common but is still observed. Chronic head lice infestations are occasionally associated with methicillin-resistant *Staphylococcus aureus* (MRSA) or nephritogenic strains of *Streptococcus* spp.,[6] either introduced by the lice themselves or by a child's scratching. Meinking[1] demonstrated *S. aureus* growth on Petri dishes traversed by head lice.

Thankfully, head lice have never been shown to transmit blood-born viral disease, such as HIV or hepatitis. However, HIV has been recovered from crab lice.[1] Head lice are close relatives to body lice, which live in the seams of clothing.[7] Body lice can transmit *Rickettsia prowazekii* (causing epidemic typhus), *Borrelia recurrentis* (causing relapsing fever), and *Bartonella quintana* (causing trench fever). Infectivity of these pathogens are thought to be from inhalation of aerosolised louse faeces, which are felt to accumulate in larger quantities in the seams of clothing than in the scalp.[3]

EPIDEMIOLOGY

Depending on the geography, the prevalence of head lice in schools ranges from 1–10% at any given time. Lice most commonly infest children aged 6–11 years, but any age group is susceptible.[8] In nearly every clinical trial done on head lice products, females are represented more than males.[8] The female predisposition might be accounted for by longer average hair length or sharing of fomites during play. Interestingly, blacks in the US and northern Europe appear to be less susceptible, but not immune, to lice infestation due to incompatible shape of the hair shaft with that of the lice claws.[8]

DIAGNOSIS

Making a diagnosis of head lice is relatively straight-forward provided that you know what you are looking for. Overdiagnosis and misdiagnosis occur by inexperienced individuals.[9] The louse eggs, or nits, are 0.8 mm in diameter.[1] An unhatched nit is brown, and a hatched nit is white (Fig. 1). Both are firmly adherent to the hair shaft, unlike flakes of dandruff, lint, or hair casts. Because lice are sensitive to dehydration and because the scalp represents a humid

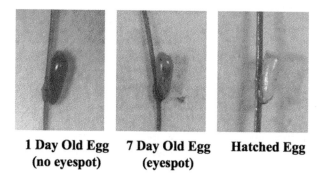

1 Day Old Egg   **7 Day Old Egg**   **Hatched Egg**
(no eyespot)   **(eyespot)**

Fig. 1 Nits: unhatched nits are brown, develop an eyespot at day 4, and appear white once hatched. Photographs courtesy of Joseph Strycharz, Department of Veterinary & Animal Science, University of Massachusetts Amherst (laboratory of Dr John Clark).

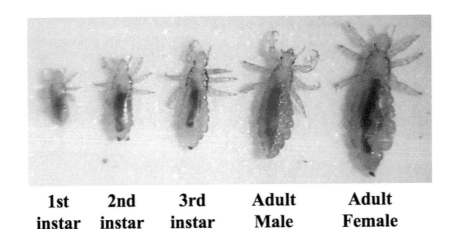

1st   2nd   3rd   Adult   Adult
instar instar instar Male   Female

Fig. 2 Head lice: the head lice shown here (in order of increasing size) are nymph, adult male, and adult female. Photographs courtesy of Joseph Strycharz, Department of Veterinary & Animal Science, University of Massachusetts Amherst (laboratory of Dr John Clark).

micro-environment for the lice, in active infestations in dry climates, viable nits would be located very near the scalp. In humid climates, viable nits can be found further away from the scalp. A live louse (Fig. 2) is about 2.1–3.3 mm long.[1] Lice can most commonly be found at the nape of the neck and behind the ears.

Signs of lice can include red papules at the site of louse bites and scalp pyoderma from superinfected bites and/or excoriations. Children infested with lice can often be observed scratching their heads. Symptoms can include pruritus; however, lice infestations are often asymptomatic.[8] The identification of nits alone presents a small dilemma. Williams *et al.*[4] demonstrated that when children in a school setting were screened for lice, of 50 children with nits alone, 18% were found to have live lice at a later examination. In the absence of prospective data on treating children based only on the presence of nits, the decision to treat a child with only nits is somewhat subjective. If a safe, effective therapy is available, there appears to be little downside to treat the child with nits alone.

Differential diagnosis

While one can make a very broad differential diagnosis of head lice on the basis of scalp pruritus or nits, there is often little question to an experienced examiner. Unfortunately, many people are inexperienced in the diagnosis. In one study where examiners sent in their suspected lice specimens to an entomology centre, doctors were correct only 17% of the time, whereas teachers were correct 86% of the time.[9] Other entities are often mistaken for nits. For example, seborrheic dermatitis produces mobile scale and often a more diffuse scalp erythema. Hair casts are easily moved along the hair shaft. Hair shaft abnormalities, such as monilethrix or trichorhexis nodosa, can be distinguished via microscopic examination, as can trichomycosis axillaris, white piedra, and black piedra. Other arthropods, such as aphids or crab lice, can be mistaken for head lice. In the case of crab lice infestation of the scalp, therapy is the same.

Table 1 Life cycle of a female head louse

Stage of life cycle	Time in each stage (days)		
	Minimum	Maximum	Average
Egg without eyespot[a]	< 1	4[b]	4[c]
Egg (lay to hatch)	7	12	8.5
First instar to egg-laying adult	8.5	11	9.7

[a]No eyespot implies the egg is not susceptible to neurotoxins.
[b]No data in head lice are available, so 4 days is an estimate.
[c]Average time cannot be calculated but is, at most, 4 days.
Adapted from Lebwohl *et al.*[5]

HEAD LICE LIFE CYCLE AND SURVIVAL

When considering head lice therapeutics, certain aspects of lice biology must be understood; specifically, their life cycle, mechanism of air transport, and ability to survive off the host. For practical purposes, three stages of the head lice life cycle can be considered: (i) egg without an eyespot; (ii) egg from lay to hatch; and (iii) newly hatched louse to egg-laying adult. Table 1 summarises times spent in each stage.

In the face of non-ovicidal anti-lice therapy, survival is favoured with the longest time as an ovum (12 days) and the shortest time from hatchling to egg-laying adult (8.5 days). Of specific significance is the development of the eye spot at day 4. The eye spot indicates the development of a nervous system and thus susceptibility to agents, such as permethrin and malathion, that act on it.[5]

Anti-lice agents can be categorised into two groups – primarily pediculicidal (and only limitedly ovicidal) or both pediculicidal and ovicidal. The 'pediculicidal only' agent requires three treatments separated by 1 week for the following reason. At day 0, all lice are killed. Eggs at all stages, but most importantly newly laid eggs and imminent hatchlings, remain. At day 7, all hatchlings are killed (but they have not had time to mature sufficiently to lay eggs). At days 13–15, eggs that are 7–12 days old remain. Hatchlings from a day 12 egg are killed with a day 13 treatment. Hatchlings from a day 7 egg will mature to egg-laying by day 15.5, making the upper limit of the timing of the third treatment to be at day 15.

The 'pediculicidal and ovicidal' agent requires two treatments separated by 7 days. At day 0, all lice and eggs with eyespots would be killed. Immature eggs would remain. At day 7, eggs without eyespots now have eyespots and would be killed. Theoretically, one could retreat at days 5–11. At day 5, a newly laid egg should have developed an eyespot. If a day 4 egg without an eyespot were treated, then it would take a minimum of three additional days to hatch and 8.5 additional days to mature to egg-laying; hence, treatment before day 11.5 would ensure eradication.[5]

Mechanism of air transport

Lice breathe via spiracles but can also obtain air via diffusion through their entire cuticle.[10] When placed under occlusive stress, such as water submersion, lice close their spiracles until the stress is removed, which explains how they

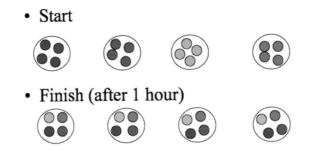

Fig. 3 Head lice transmission experiment: 20 each of lice painted four different colours were placed on four sisters' heads (one colour per head). The children slept next to each other in a hammock. After 1 h, all four heads harboured all four colours of lice.

can survive up to 16 h under water submersion.[11] When faced with occlusive stress from white petrolatum, lice will force the spiracles open much like one blows a stuffy nose.[10] Recent systems using 50% isopropyl myristate are being formulated that claim to disrupt the louse cuticle, resulting in fatal dehydration of the louse. It is unclear if such therapy will be uniformly effective, if it will kill nits, and how often it would have to be repeated.

Ability to survive off the host

Lice have been shown to survive off the human host for up to 55 h (mean, 21 h), during which time they can re-infest.[12] Lice can be found on pillow cases of infested individuals, albeit uncommonly.[13] The implication for environmental treatment is to vacuum furniture and launder bed sheets in a dryer. While nits can likely survive for 12 days off the host, the likelihood that the host is present upon their hatching while off the host (say, on a stuffed animal) is slim. Therefore, non-launderable fomites are best kept in a bag for 3 days to ensure desiccation of lice (with deliberate lack of concern for nits).

Transmission

The primary mode of lice transmission is head-to-head contact. This is best demonstrated by a study done by Terri Meinking[1] in which she collected 80 lice, tagged four groups of 20 lice with different colour fluorescent dyes, and placed 20 of any one colour on the heads of each of four siblings (see Fig. 3). After 1 h of sleeping in the same hammock, all heads had all colours of lice.[1] Head lice are host-specific, so they are not transmitted to or from pets. Lice do not jump or fly, but rather crawl quickly from scalp to scalp. Indeed, they can move up to 30 cm/min.[1]

THERAPIES

Head lice therapies can be subdivided into ovicidal and pediculicidal versus pediculicidal only. Of each of these, there are chemical and physical methods. Table 2 summarises the modalities.

CHEMICAL METHODS

Of the chemical methods, all (except trimethoprim/sulfamethoxazole) are neurotoxic in one way or another to the head louse, leading to paralysis and

Table 2 Head lice therapies

Modality	Pyrethroids, pyrethrins, ± piperonyl butoxide
Therapy	Chemical, pediculicidal. In the absence of resistance, pyrethroids are ovicidal as well
Safety concerns	Rare: asthma in those allergic to ragweed; possible link to leukaemia
Efficacy	Resistance is wide-spread; infestivity is a problem between treatments
Modality	Malathion
Therapy	Chemical, pediculicidal, ovicidal
Safety concerns	Flammable when vehicle is isopropyl alcohol
Efficacy	Resistance is wide-spread, but not in the US; best in combination with isopropyl alcohol and terpineol
Modality	Lindane
Therapy	Chemical, pediculicidal
Safety concerns	Seizures; water pollution
Efficacy	Resistance is wide-spread; infestivity is a problem between treatments
Modality	Carbaryl
Therapy	Chemical, pediculicidal, ovicidal
Safety concerns	Theoretically carcinogenic, but not proven
Efficacy	Occasional resistance has been reported
Modality	Benzyl benzoate
Therapy	Chemical, pediculicidal. Data as to ovicidality are not available
Safety concerns	Unknown
Efficacy	Unknown
Modality	Ivermectin
Therapy	Chemical, pediculicidal
Safety concerns	Hepatotoxicity; seizures in younger patients
Efficacy	Not effective as single dose orally; scant evidence supports topical therapy
Modality	Trimethoprim/sulfamethoxazole
Therapy	Chemical, pediculicidal
Safety concerns	Severe drug rash (Stevens Johnson syndrome); bacterial antibiotic resistance
Efficacy	No theoretical basis to support its use; clinical evidence for efficacy is conflicting
Modality	Terpineol (in tea tree oil)
Therapy	Chemical, pediculicidal, ovicidal
Safety concerns	Rare: allergic contact dermatitis
Efficacy	Effective in combination with malathion; as monotherapy, only scant evidence
Modality	Isopropyl myristate 50%
Therapy	Physical, pediculicidal
Safety concerns	None
Efficacy	Efficacy remains to be validated in larger clinical trials; infestivity is a problem between treatments
Modality	Dimethicone
Therapy	Physical, pediculicidal
Safety concerns	None
Efficacy	Efficacy appears to be less than malathion but greater than Bug Busting; infestivity is a problem between treatments
Modality	Cetaphil liquid cleanser
Therapy	Physical, pediculicidal
Safety concerns	Not rigorously studied
Efficacy	Clinical study was open label with no control group and not independently validated; infestivity is a problem between treatments

Table 2 *(continued)* Head lice therapies

Modality	Nit combing or Bug Busting
Therapy	Physical, neither pediculicidal nor ovicidal
Safety concerns	Pain due to hair pulling
Efficacy	Studies have shown a 60% efficacy at best combing four separate days for up to 13 days; infestivity is a problem between treatments
Modality	Shaving the head
Therapy	Physical, neither pediculicidal nor ovicidal
Safety concerns	Negative psychosocial impact
Efficacy	No formal efficacy studies exist, but lice require hair shafts to lay eggs and to stay on the scalp
Modality	Mayonnaise, olive oil
Therapy	Physical, neither pediculicidal nor ovicidal
Safety concerns	Bacterial overgrowth
Efficacy	Not effective
Modality	Vinegar
Therapy	Physical, neither pediculicidal nor ovicidal
Safety concerns	Burning of scalp
Efficacy	Not effective
Modality	Kerosene
Therapy	Chemical, neither pediculicidal nor ovicidal
Safety concerns	Possible carcinogen, flammable
Efficacy	Not effective
Modality	Petroleum jelly
Therapy	Physical, pediculicidal, ovicidal
Safety concerns	Safe, but difficult to remove and messy
Efficacy	Efficacy in one *in vitro* study showed 94% ovicidality and 62% pediculicidality
Modality	Water submersion
Therapy	Physical, neither pediculicidal nor ovicidal
Safety concerns	None
Efficacy	Not effective

death by dehydration. As such, efficacy occurs when the louse has a developed nervous system. Hence, an ovum younger than 4 days old will be unaffected by these agents. Agents that are non-ovicidal, presumably by failing to penetrate or disrupt the egg, require three treatments separated by 1 week. Agents of this nature, such as permethrin and lindane, are labelled by the governments that approved them for two treatments. That is, there is a discrepancy between labelled application times and those dictated by the head louse life cycle.[5]

Chemical agents act via selective toxicity to the louse over the human. Therefore, the stigma that such agents receive in the lay press as 'poisons that should be avoided at all costs' is unwarranted when used topically, except perhaps for lindane. Each molecule will be considered in turn.

Lindane (γ-benzene hexachloride), an organochlorine

Mode of action: Lindane non-competitively inhibits the γ-amino butyric acid (GABA) receptor, which typically binds GABA, an inhibitory neurotransmitter. Neuronal hyperstimulation results in paralysis.

Mode of resistance: Mutations in the GABA-receptor gene cause decreased affinity for lindane.

Toxicity: Potential neurotoxicity, including seizures and death, has been reported rarely after labelled use and more so with repeat treatments.[14] Patients weighing less than 110 lb are most at risk. Lindane persists in fat and in the environment.[15] One bottle of lindane can pollute 6 million gallons of water and cost up to US$4000 to clean up.[16]

Comment: Lindane should be applied only for 4 min and for a single treatment, not to be repeated. Because it is pediculicidal only, the head lice life cycle calls for three weekly treatments, which is unsafe. *In vitro* data also suggest 4 min is too short.[17] In the light of other safer, more effective, and environmentally friendlier options, lindane should rarely, if ever, be used.

Malathion, an organophosphate

Mode of action: In the louse, malathion is converted to malaoxon, which non-competitively inhibits acetylcholinesterase, resulting in neuronal hyperexcitation and louse paralysis.

Mode of resistance: Increased levels of carboxylesterases (resulting in either sequestration or catabolism), decreased sensitivity of acetylcholinesterase to malaoxon, or elevated metabolism of malathion by cytochrome P450 monooxygenases, glutathione-S-transferases, and phosphotriesterases may account for malathion resistance in head lice.[5]

Toxicity: Due to rapid conversion of malathion by plasma carboxylesterases to non-toxic metabolites in mammals, including humans, pure, pharmaceutical-grade malathion is very safe. Danger occurs when malathion containing isomalathion impurities is used or when high concentrations of malathion are used (as may be the case with agricultural-grade malathion). Isomalathion inhibits plasma carboxylesterases, preventing malathion's detoxification. The liver would then convert malathion to malaoxon, which would inhibit acetylcholinesterase. When malathion is contained in an isopropyl alcoholic vehicle, the mixture is flammable. However, no reports of bodily injury exist due to burns from such formulations' catching fire. If ingested, the isopropyl alcohol, much more so than the small amount of malathion, can cause respiratory depression.[5]

Comment: Malathion, specifically formulated in combination with terpineol and isopropyl alcohol, enjoys nearly complete efficacy, no resistance to date, and an excellent safety profile. It is both ovicidal and pediculicidal. Indeed, British lice that were malathion-resistant were susceptible to the combination.[18] In clinical studies, often only one application was all that was needed. The presence of isopropyl alcohol may account for single application cures due to denaturation of potein in the shells of nits both with and without eyespots. A second application at 1 week is safe and increases the likelihood of cure.[5] This application regimen also corresponds to that which is dictated by the head louse life cycle.

Permethrin and pyrethrins

Nomenclature: Pyrethrums originate from *Chrysanthemum cineriaefolium*. Pyrethrins are the insecticidal fraction of pyrethrums. Permethrin is a pyrethroid, which denotes a synthetic pyrethrin.[5]

Mode of action: Pyrethrins and permethrin bind to voltage-gated sodium channels in the louse, causing delayed neuronal repolarisation, followed by neuronal hyperexcitability, and subsequent paralysis.[5]

Mode of resistance: Lice have developed double mutations in the voltage-gated sodium channel (termed knock-down resistance or kdr) that decrease the channel's affinity for pyrethrins or permethrin.[19] A higher concentration of permethrin (*e.g.*, 5% used for scabies) is unlikely to overcome this decreased receptor affinity. Lice have also evolved a higher capacity to metabolise pyrethrins via up-regulated microsomal enzyme activity. As such, pipernoyl butoxide is often added to pyrethrin preparations to inhibit these microsomal enzymes allowing for an increased half-life of pyrethrins in the louse.[5]

Toxicity: Human voltage-gated channels are not susceptible to pyrethrins or permethrin, making these compounds particularly safe. Rare cases of asthma exacerbation in ragweed allergic patients have been reported with natural pyrethrins. Very high doses of permethrin can theoretically induce leukaemia by causing a translocation in the mixed-lineage leukaemia (MLL) gene.[20]

Comment: Due to the high prevalence of the kdr gene mutations in lice populations world-wide, the utility of pyrethrins and permethrin in head lice is waning.[5] Package inserts of products containing permethrin and pyrethrins frequently call for one to two applications; this schedule is less than the three applications suggested by the head lice life cycle for non-ovicidal treatments. Treatment with these agents still can be considered as reasonable first steps (indeed, permethrin is ovicidal in the absence of resistance), but one must acknowledge the risk of continued infestivity both with failed treatment and between treatments.

Carbaryl, a carbamate

Mode of action: Carbaryl competitively inhibits acetylcholinesterase, resulting in neuronal hyperexcitation and louse paralysis.

Mode of resistance: Resistance to this compound has only infrequently been reported. In other insects, carbaryl resistance occurs via altered binding sites of acetylcholinesterase and/or increased oxidative metabolism of carbaryl.[21]

Toxicity: Theoretical concerns of carcinogenicity have been raised, causing the UK Government to change the status of carbaryl from over-the-counter to prescription.

Comment: Like malathion, carbaryl appears to be a safe and effective option for head lice. Data on *in vitro* ovicidal and pediculicidal rates in head lice are lacking, but small *in vivo* clinical trials suggest excellent efficacy with two applications separated by 1 week.[22–24] As these trials were performed over two decades ago, it is unclear what effect the development of resistance has had on the present-day efficacy of carbaryl.

Benzyl benzoate

Mode of action: The mechanism of action is unknown.

Mode of resistance: It is unclear if head lice resistance to benzyl benzoate exists.

Toxicity: Toxicity data are not available to render a valid assessment of its safety profile.

Comment: There is a lack of data on the safety and efficacy of this product for head lice. The available formulation in the UK contains terpineol,[25] which may contribute to its efficacy. In the absence of known ovicidal and pediculicidal rates in head lice, it is unclear if two or three treatments would be required (as dictated by the head lice life cycle).

Ivermectin, an avermectin

Mode of action: Ivermectin selectively binds to glutamate-gated chloride ion channels in invertebrate nerve and muscle cells, causing hyperexcitability and paralysis.

Mode of resistance: It is unclear if head lice are resistant to ivermectin.

Toxicity: Orally, ivermectin can occasionally cause elevated liver transaminases; more importantly, it can cross an immature blood–brain barrier, such that dosing in children is not recommended.

Comment: Since ivermectin is administered orally to the human host, only hatched lice feeding on human blood can be affected; therefore, it is pediculicidal only. As such, three doses separated by 1 week apart would be required. There is a lack of safety or efficacy data to support such a dosing schedule, especially in children.

Trimethoprim/sulfamethoxazole

Mode of action: This combination is thought to kill symbiotic bacteria in the head louse gut that are thought to provide essential B vitamins to the louse; however, some argue that head lice symbiotes cannot synthesise B vitamins, calling into question the theoretical benefit of this therapy.[1]

Mode of resistance: Bacterial resistance to the combination would render this therapy ineffective.

Toxicity: Severe drug hypersensitivity, including Stevens Johnson syndrome, and antibiotic resistance are the major problems with this therapy.

Comment: The two largest studies examining the efficacy of trimethoprim/sulfamethoxazole yield conflicting conclusions as to the combination's efficacy in lice. Hipolito *et al.*[26] found a benefit, and Sim *et al.*[27] showed no benefit. Dosing is complicated by a lack of knowledge of how long it takes the drug to kill the gut symbiotes. It is pediculicidal only, if at all. In the light of poor evidence for efficacy, risk of drug hypersensitivity, and risk of inducing drug resistance in an era of MRSA that is otherwise still susceptible to trimethoprim/sulfamethoxazole, this therapy should be reserved for only the most refractory cases of lice.

Terpineol (found in tea tree oil), a terpenoid

Mode of action: Terpineol inhibits acetylcholinesterase and binds octopamine receptors, causing neuronal hyperactivity and death in insects.[28]

Mode of resistance: Resistance to terpineol has not been demonstrated in head lice to date.

Toxicity: Human toxicity of terpineol is not well-studied, such that data are not available to provide guidance. Allergic contact dermatitis to terpineol has been reported.[29]

Comment: Terpineol has been demonstrated *in vitro* to kill lice and eggs, albeit not 100% of the time.[30] As such, it is sub-optimal as monotherapy. In combination with malathion, and possibly with other agents, terpineol is an excellent adjunct to topical lice therapy.[18]

PHYSICAL METHODS

Physical modalities to treat head lice include suffocation of the louse (but not necessarily the egg), disruption of the louse cuticle causing dehydration, or lice and nit removal either by combing or shaving. The commonly used physical methods are considered below.

Isopropyl myristate 50% in 50% ST-cyclomethicone

Mode of action: Isopropyl myristate is purported to dissolve the waxy coat of the louse exoskeleton, causing fatal dehydration of the louse. As the louse eggshell is proteinaceous, this chemical is not expected to kill eggs.

Comment: In the isopropyl myristate arm of one small randomised trial, only 18 of 30 subjects were cured at 21 days by an intention-to-treat analysis. Three treatments would be necessary were this agent perfectly pediculicidal; however, as the data demonstrate, this agent is imperfect.[31] Isopropyl myristate does provide an alternative for those phobic of conventional chemical modalities.

Dimethicone 4% in cyclomethicone

Mode of action: Dimethicone is reported to coat head lice, both immobilising the lice and interfering with their ability to manage water.[32]

Comment: Dimethicone is available in a variety of over-the-counter preparations. Efficacy rates of one 4% dimethicone preparation was 70% with no significant side effects.[32] Dimethicone appears to be pediculicidal only, such that three applications are dictated by the head lice life cycle. Infestivity between treatments remains a problem.

Cetaphil liquid cleanser

Mode of action: Cetaphil liquid cleanser is reported to coat the louse with the wet material and permanently contract around it when dried with a hair drier.[33]

Comment: Three applications at weekly intervals are recommended. This schedule corresponds with the head lice life cycle. Physical removal of nits is required. While excellent results have been reported, the initial studies were open-label and independently performed confirming studies are lacking.

Bug Busting (as representative of nit removal)

Mode of action: The hair is wet with water, then a specially designed, fine-tooth nit comb is used to comb out lice and nits systematically in four sessions spaced evenly over 13 days.[34]

Comment: This method has a cure rate at best of about 60%[35] and is often painful, time consuming, and subject to human error and lack of rigor. Infestivity between treatments is also a problem. Related nit removal services, whereby someone comes to the home to do combing and house cleaning for the family, can be quite expensive and has never been validated. For those averse to chemical treatments, however, this option is reasonable so long as the user is aware that cure rates are far from absolute.

Folk remedies – *e.g.*, kerosene, vinegar, mayonnaise, melted butter, petroleum jelly

Mode of action: None of the mechanisms of actions of these treatments have been experimentally validated. Kerosene is thought to poison the louse.

Vinegar is thought to dissolve the nit casing, louse cuticle, and nit cement. Mayonnaise, melted butter, and petroleum jelly are felt to occlude the lice. All these therapies have been examined *in vitro*. None were reliably effective, perhaps with the exception of petroleum jelly, which was able to kill eggs 94% of the time and lice 62% of the time.[11]

Managing contacts

Of equal importance to choosing the proper therapy for any one individual found to have lice is to identify and treat close contacts who may also have the infestation. By doing so, a cycle of infestation and re-infestation can be avoided. Those at highest risk are household members, frequent visitors to the household, and close friends. Less likely, but still at risk enough to warrant screening, are classroom contacts.

Because lice are difficult to detect, one reasonable approach is to treat empirically those at highest risk with screening of class-mates. Conversely, some healthcare providers and parents disfavour potential unnecessary exposure to therapy unless a definitive infestation has been identified. Fortunately, the majority of first-line therapies, such as malathion, carbaryl, petroleum jelly, or nit combing, are extremely safe.

Managing the environment

As mentioned above, bedding and any clothes (including hats, jackets, and scarves) worn by the patient should be placed in a dryer for 10 min at 60°C. Hair brushes can be placed in hot (60°C or more) water for 10 min. Fomites, such as stuffed animals, that cannot be laundered should be placed in a bag for 3 days. Rugs, chairs, and couches should be vacuumed. Fumigation or spraying of the home with permethrin or other insecticides is not necessary.

SCHOOL POLICY

Whether or not to exclude a child from school is a hotly debated issue. Common sense and science dictate that 'no nit' policies in schools harm the child and society and do little to prevent transmission of lice. However, the teachers and nurses that deal personally with a lice-infested child experience the same visceral disgust as most people do when faced with someone who has lice. Specifically, the urge and instinct is to keep them away. It is our job as part of the healthcare community to educate school personnel about lice transmission, identification, and treatment so as to quell their fears and concerns and dispel their misconceptions about lice. As such, we can make school personnel truly believe that 'no nit' policies are wrong and feel comfortable with the management of their students with lice.

Key points for clinical practice

- Head lice should be treated because of their negative psychosocial impact and the pruritus they cause.
- Because hair grows 1 cm/month and lice lay eggs near the scalp, eggs found 2 cm from the scalp represents a 2-month-old infestation.

(cont'd)

Key points for clinical practice (cont'd)

- Lice can be diagnosed by finding nits adherent to the hair shaft and (preferably) live lice, both most commonly located at the nape of the neck and behind the ears.

- Lice can survive off the host for up to 55 h. Implications are to keep non-launderable items in a bag for 3 days to kill stray lice.

- Lice are exquisitely sensitive to dehydration. Implications are to place launderable items, such as bedding and hats, in a dryer at 60°C for at least 10 min to kill stray lice and eggs.

- The primary mode of lice transmission is head-to-head contact.

- Pertinent features of the head lice life cycle are: egg develops eyespot (*i.e.*, a nervous system) at day 4, hatches at the latest by day 12, and is able to lay eggs as soon as day 7 after hatching. That is, non-ovicidal therapies will not kill a viable nit at the traditionally suggested 7-day re-application time of most pediculicides.

- Non-ovicidal pediculicides require three treatments separated by 1 week. Therapies that are both pediculicidal and ovicidal require two treatments separated by 1 week.

- Choice of therapy must balance safety, efficacy, and regional resistance patterns of the lice.

- At the time of writing, the most effective therapy (ovicidal and pediculicidal) for head lice appears to be malathion formulated in isopropyl alcohol with terpineol. Carbaryl is a reasonable alternative.

- For those averse to agents that act on the louse nervous system, Bug Busting, isopropyl myristate 50%, petrolatum, and Cetaphil cleanser are possible alternatives. Shaving the head should be reserved for extreme cases.

- Resistance to permethrin and pyrethrins has rendered these safe therapies somewhat unreliable.

- Lindane is potentially toxic, persists in the environment, and lice have developed resistance to it. As such, it should not be used.

- Contacts of index cases, including classmates, should be screened. Consider empiric therapy for close household contacts, particularly if they share a bed.

- Fumigation or spraying of the home is not necessary; however, vacuuming furniture and carpets may have some validity.

- Excluding children from school due to head lice (the 'no-nit policy') is hurtful to the child, the parents, and the school and does little to prevent lice transmission.

ACKNOWLEDGEMENTS

Conflict of interest statement: the author is a vice president of Taro Pharmaceuticals U.S.A., Inc. and a major shareholder of Taro Pharmaceutical Industries, Ltd (Taro). Taro manufactures and sells Ovide® (malathion) Lotion, 0.5%.

References

1. Meinking TL. Infestations. *Curr Probl Dermatol* 1999; **11**: 73–118.
2. Mumcuoglu KY. Head lice in drawings of kindergarten children. *Isr J Psychiatry Relat Sci* 1991; **28**: 25–32.
3. Maunder JW. The appreciation of lice. *R Inst Gr B* 1984; **55**: 1–31.
4. Williams LK, Reichert A, MacKenzie WR, Hightower AW, Blake PA. Lice, nits, and school policy. *Pediatrics* 2001; **107**: 1011–1015.
5. Lebwohl M, Clark L, Levitt J. Therapy for head lice based on life cycle, resistance, and safety considerations. *Pediatrics* 2007; **119**: 965–974.
6. Mumcuoglu KY, Klaus S, Kafka D, Teiler M, Miller J. Clinical observations related to head lice infestation. *J Am Acad Dermatol* 1991; **25**: 248–251.
7. Light JE, Toups MA, Reed DL. What's in a name: the taxonomic status of human head and body lice. *Mol Phylogenet Evol* 2008; **47**: 1203–1216.
8. Burgess IF. Human lice and their management. *Adv Parasitol* 1995; **36**: 271–342.
9. Pollack RJ, Kiszewski AE, Spielman A. Overdiagnosis and consequent mismanagement of head louse infestations in North America. *Pediatr Infect Dis J* 2000; **19**: 689–693.
10. Burkhart CG, Burkhart CN. Asphyxiation of lice with topical agents, not a reality...yet. *J Am Acad Dermatol* 2006; **54**: 721–722.
11. Takano-Lee M, Edman JD, Mullens BA, Clark JM. Home remedies to control head lice: assessment of home remedies to control the human head louse, *Pediculus humanus capitis* (Anoplura: Pediculidae). *J Pediatr Nurs* 2004; **19**: 393–398.
12. Chunge RN, Scott FE, Underwood JE, Zavarella KJ. A pilot study to investigate transmission of headlice. *Can J Public Health* 1991; **82**: 207–208.
13. Speare R, Cahill C, Thomas G. Head lice on pillows, and strategies to make a small risk even less. *Int J Dermatol* 2003; **42**: 626–629.
14. Lindane Package Insert, Morton Grove Pharmaceuticals, Inc., Morton Grove, IL and Alliant Pharmaceuticals, Inc., Alpharetta, GA, USA. June 2005.
15. Kutz FW, Wood PH, Bottimore DP. Organochlorine pesticides and polychlorinated biphenyls in human adipose tissue. *Rev Environ Contam Toxicol* 1991; **120**: 1–82.
16. Water Policy Report via InsideEPA.com, Inside Washington Publishers, 2007; 16(1).
17. Meinking TL, Entzel P, Villar ME *et al*. Comparative efficacy of treatments for *Pediculosis capitis* infestations: update 2000. *Arch Dermatol* 2001; **137**: 287–292.
18. Downs AM, Narayan S, Stafford KA, Coles GC. Effectiveness of Ovide against malathion-resistant head lice. *Arch Dermatol* 2005; **141**: 1318.
19. Lee SH, Yoon KS, Williamson MS *et al*. Molecular analysis of kdr-like resistance in permethrin-resistant strains of head lice, *Pediculosis capitis*. *Pestic Biochem Physiol* 2000; **66**: 130–143.
20. Borkhardt A, Wilda M, Fuchs U, Gortner L, Reiss I. Congenital leukemia after heavy abuse of permethrin during pregnancy. *Arch Dis Child* 2003; **88**: F436–F437.
21. Downs AM, Stafford KA, Hunt LP, Ravenscroft JC, Coles GC. Widespread insecticide resistance in head lice to the over-the-counter pediculocides in England, and the emergence of carbaryl resistance. *Br J Dermatol* 2002; **146**: 88–93.
22. Armoni M, Bibi H, Schlesinger M, Pollak S, Metzker A. *Pediculosis capitis*: why prefer a solution to shampoo or spray? *Pediatr Dermatol* 1988; **5**: 273–275.
23. Donaldson RJ, Logie S. Comparative trial of shampoos for treatment of head infestation. *J R Soc Health* 1986; **106**: 39–40.
24. Preston S. An assessment of two carbaryl preparations. *R Soc Health J* 1979; **99**: 173.
25. Ascabiol® Emulsion 25%w/v. Aventis. May 2006.
<http://emc.medicines.org.uk/emc/assets/c/html/DisplayDoc.asp?format=original&documentid=3111> [Accessed 26 May 2008].

26. Hipolito RB, Mallorca FG, Zuniga-Macaraiq ZO, Apolinario PC, Wheeler-Sherman J. Head lice infestation: single drug versus combination therapy with one percent permethrin and trimethoprim/sulfamethoxazole. *Pediatrics* 2001; **107**: E30.

27. Sim S, Lee IY, Lee KJ *et al*. A survey on head lice infestation in Korea (2001) and the therapeutic efficacy of oral trimethoprim/sulfamethoxazole adding to lindane shampoo. *Korean J Parasitol* 2003; **41**: 57–61.

28. Enan E. Insecticidal activity of essential oils: octopaminergic sites of action. *Comp Biochem Physiol C Toxicol Pharmacol* 2001; **130**: 325–337.

29. Cachao P, Menezes Brandao F, Carmo M, Frazao S, Silva M. Allergy to oil of turpentine in Portugal. *Contact Dermatitis* 1986; **14**: 205–208.

30. Yang YC, Choi HY, Choi WS, Clark JM, Ahn YJ. Ovicidal and adulticidal activity of *Eucalyptus globulus* leaf oil terpenoids against *Pediculus humanus capitis* (Anoplura: Pediculidae). *J Agric Food Chem* 2004; **52**: 2507–2511.

31. Kaul N, Palma KG, Silagy SS, Goodman JJ, Toole J. North American efficacy and safety of a novel pediculicide rinse, isopropyl myristate 50% (Resultz). *J Cutan Med Surg* 2007; **11**: 161–167.

32. Burgess IF, Brown CM, Lee PN. Treatment of head louse infestation with 4% dimeticone lotion: randomised controlled equivalence trial. *BMJ* 2005; **330**: 1423.

33. Pearlman DL. A simple treatment for head lice: dry-on, suffocation-based pediculicide. *Pediatrics* 2004; **114**: e275–e279.

34. Bingham P, Kirk S, Hill N, Figueroa J. The methodology and operation of a pilot randomized control trial of the effectiveness of the Bug Busting method against a single application insecticide product for head louse treatment. *Public Health* 2000; **114**: 265–268.

35. Hill N, Moor G, Cameron MM *et al*. Single blind, randomised, comparative study of the Bug Buster kit and over the counter pediculicide treatments against head lice in the United Kingdom. *BMJ* 2005; **331**: 384–387.

Tonse N.K. Raju Jill V. Hunter Karin B. Nelson

8

Ischaemic perinatal stroke

Ischaemic perinatal stroke is a major cause of neurological and developmental disability. It is the most common known cause of cerebral palsy.[1-8] With increasing use of advanced magnetic resonance imaging (MRI) techniques, this condition is being diagnosed with greater frequency. This chapter provides a brief review of ischaemic perinatal stroke.

DEFINITION

There is no precise, or universally agreed upon, definition and classification of perinatal stroke, in part due to some unique features of strokes in the perinatal period (Table 1). In this chapter, we define an ischaemic perinatal stroke as 'a neurological dysfunction due to an acute or subacute vascular ischemic event during the fetal life through 28 days of postnatal age, traditionally known as the perinatal period'.[4] This definition includes rare cases of ischaemic lesions leading to strokes in preterm infants,[9,10] fetal strokes,[11,12] and thrombosis and infarction of large cerebral venous sinuses.[13,14] It excludes brain pathology from hypoxic ischaemic encephalopathy, strokes complicating cerebral

Tonse N.K. Raju MD DCH (for correspondence)
Program Scientist/Medical Officer, Pregnancy and Perinatology Branch, *Eunice Kennedy Shriver* National Institute of Child Health and Human Development, National Institutes of Health, 6100 Executive Blvd, Room 4B03, Bethesda, MD 20892-MS7510, USA
E-mail: rajut@mail.nih.gov

Jill V. Hunter MBBS
Baylor College of Medicine and Texas Children's Hospital, Houston, Texas, USA

Karin B. Nelson MD
National Institute of Neurological Disorders and Stroke, National Institutes of Health, Bethesda, Maryland, USA and Department of Neurology, Children's National Medical Center, Washington DC, USA

Table 1 Some unique features of perinatal stroke

Timing and incidence

- Stroke can occur at any time from fetal life through 28 days of postnatal age, but a majority is thought to occur 3 days before or after birth
- The precise timing of perinatal stroke is very difficult to establish
- Strokes are 17 times more common during the perinatal period than later in childhood

Aetiology

- In most cases, the aetiology remains undetermined
- The sources of pathology can be in the mother, the fetus/newborn, or the placenta
- Because of high fetal haemoglobin and low sickle haemoglobin concentrations in the neonatal period, sickle cell anaemia is not a cause of ischaemic perinatal stroke
- In non-twin sibships, it is very rare to see more than one sibling affected, indicating a greater role for environmental factors than genetic factors in the causal pathway
- The most common associated factors are inherited and acquired thrombotic, and inherited and acquired autoimmune conditions in the mother, the fetus, or the newborn. However, most women and their infants with such conditions remain healthy
- Because of the patency of the ductus arteriosus and foramen ovale in the perinatal period, emboli from the fetal venous circulation or from the fetal side of the placenta can cross into the arterial circulation, resulting in fetal/neonatal ischaemic cerebral stroke

Pathology

- Arterial ischaemia is the most common pathology, followed by sinovenous thrombosis. The left middle cerebral artery followed by the right are the most commonly affected vessels
- Distinction between a cerebral haemorrhagic lesion and an ischaemic infarction can be difficult, since an ischaemic lesion can become haemorrhagic and a haematoma can lead to vascular occlusion and infarction
- The size of the pathological lesion may be disproportionate to the severity of signs and symptoms
- Affected infants may have other systemic thromobo-emboli

Diagnosis

- Advanced MRI techniques are the only definitive means of establishing a diagnosis in the living patient.

---

vascular malformations, intra- and periventricular haemorrhage, periventricular leukomalacia, and other forms of white matter lesions seen most often in preterm infants.

Synonymous terms

Other terms used to describe ischaemic perinatal strokes with minor modifications in the definitional criteria are: arterial ischaemic stroke, perinatal arterial stroke; early and late neonatal stroke, perinatal ischaemic stroke and presumed perinatal stroke.[4]

CLASSIFICATION

One approach to the classification of ischaemic perinatal stroke is based on the age at diagnosis, since the precise timing of the vascular event causing stroke usually cannot be determined, and the nature of cerebral pathology may be difficult to discern even after neuro-imaging studies or pathological examination. The following categories have been suggested:[4]

1. **Fetal stroke**: a stroke diagnosed in the fetal period using imaging studies or, in cases of stillbirths, with the help of an autopsy. Although strokes can occur at any time during fetal life, a diagnosis of fetal stroke is usually made after 20 weeks of pregnancy.[2,4,11,12]

2. **Neonatal stroke**: a stroke diagnosed using radiographic methods (or autopsy) in the immediate newborn period, or before the completion of 28 days of age.[5]

3. **Sinovenous infarctions**: a stroke in the perinatal period associated with thrombosis of one or more major cerebral venous sinuses (straight sinus; sigmoid sinus; transverse sinus, or jugular sinus).[13,14]

4. **Presumed perinatal stroke**: an asymptomatic ischaemic stroke presumed to have occurred during the perinatal period, but diagnosed later in infancy or childhood.[15]

INCIDENCE AND SCOPE

Ischaemic stroke is more common in the perinatal period than later infancy or childhood, or at any subsequent time until late adult life. Other thrombo-embolic events also concentrate in the perinatal period.[16] Diagnosis in the living patient is by neuro-imaging, and the reported incidence in epidemiological studies and systematic reviews has varied with the frequency of neuro-imaging, especially MRI. Thus, the reported incidence has ranged between 1 in 1600 births to 1 in 5000 births.[2,5,8,9] The actual incidence is likely to be higher, since nearly one-third of affected infants remain asymptomatic in the neonatal period, only to be diagnosed later. In some cases, a diagnosis may be missed altogether. Some studies report only unilateral strokes, although one-third of strokes manifesting in the neonatal period are bilateral.[17] In a busy perinatal centre serving a region with 15,000 deliveries, one may encounter 10 infants with ischaemic perinatal stroke each year.

AETIOLOGY AND RISK FACTORS

Many factors in the mother, the fetus and newborn, and the placenta have been associated with ischaemic perinatal stroke (Table 2).[18–33]

Normal pregnancy and fetal life

Pregnancy is a recognised 'natural prothrombotic state' with an increased tendency for clot formation due to higher concentrations of fibrinogen, factors VII, VIII, X, and the von Willebrand factor; and a decreased effectiveness of anti-coagulation factors due to decreased concentrations of protein S, and

Table 2 Maternal and fetal conditions associated with perinatal stroke

Maternal conditions
- Infertility and its treatment
- Pre-eclampsia
- Prolonged rupture of membrane (> 24 h)
- Chorio-amnionitis and/or maternal infections
- Maternal autoimmune conditions and autoantibodies (platelet alloantigen-1)
- Antiphospholipid antibodies
- Placental thrombotic vasculopathy, inflammation, and other pathologies
- Dehydration
- Maternal cocaine abuse; codeine abuse
- Over-the-counter herbal supplements (*e.g.* blue-cohosh)

Abnormal haematological and thrombophilia screening tests (mother or infant)
- Activated protein C resistance factor V G1691A (factor V Leiden)
- Protein C activity/antigen prothrombin G20210A
- Free and total protein S antigen
- Antithrombin activity/antigen
- Lipoprotein (a)
- Fasting homocysteine
- 5,10-methylenetetrahydrofolate reductase (MTHFR) C677T mutation
- Lupus anticoagulant/antiphospholipid antibodies
- Fibrinogen (Clauss)
- Plasminogen
- Factor VIIIC

Fetal and/or neonatal conditions
- A history of reduced fetal movements late in pregnancy
- Large and small for gestational age with or without intra-uterine growth restriction
- Twin-to-twin transfusion syndrome
- Abnormal fetal heart rate patterns
- Mutations in procollagen IVa1
- Fetal/neonatal polycythaemia
- Congenital heart disease
- Neonatal hypoglycaemia (in preterm infants)
- Persistent fetal circulation and extracorporeal membrane oxygenation therapy
- Fetal/neonatal infections and meningitis
- Intravascular catheter-related complications
- Intra and extra cardiac thrombus formation

Non-specific
- Male infant
- Race/ethnicity (higher in African-American infants)

increased resistance to activated protein C. These changes may have an evolutionary basis to prevent excessive postpartum haemorrhage. However, they may also lead to increased cerebral (and other) infarctions. Strokes clustered around the time of delivery have been reported in 67 per 100,000 term births in the mothers – more than at any other period in a woman's life.[34]

Placenta

Properties of the placenta in ischaemic perinatal stroke are summarised in Table 3. Histopathological examination of the placenta can be of vital importance to find the cause of ischaemic perinatal stroke. Policies should be developed for proper handling and preserving of all placentas and umbilical

Table 3 Placenta in ischaemic perinatal stroke

Pathology
- Thrombotic and inflammatory lesions in the region of large umbilical cord vessels
- Evidence of disturbed uteroplacental circulation
- Perivillous fibrin deposition and ischaemic changes in placental villi
- Chronic villitis characterised by focal areas of inflammation with mononuclear cells and areas of fibrinoid necrosis

Mechanism
- Global impairment of placental function leading to hypoxia and acidosis
- Release of inflammatory mediators promoting fetal coagulopathy
- Formation of placental vascular thrombi, embolising through the patent ductus venosus or the foramen ovale
- Generation of severe fetal inflammatory responses

---

cords, since such specimens can be invaluable for later examination in fetal and neonatal stroke, presumed perinatal stroke, unexplained fetal or neonatal death, and in medicolegal cases.[35,36]

Infection
Pregnancy is also a pro-inflammatory state, increasing the potential for thrombotic interactions between inflammatory and coagulation pathways. Thus chorio-amnionitis and other infections during pregnancy are the reported risk factors for ischaemic perinatal strokes, as they can promote thrombotic episodes in the placenta, or in maternal or fetal circulation.

Acquired and inherited autoimmune and thrombotic conditions
A large number of associated thrombotic and immunological risk factors (Table 2) can enhance clot formation in the maternal or fetal vasculature, or in the uteroplacental unit. Due to the patency of the ductus arteriosus and the foramen ovale in the perinatal period, thrombi from the fetal venous circulation or the fetal side of the placenta can lead to embolisation in the fetal cerebral arterial circulation.

Maternal drug abuse and use of over-the-counter herbal preparations
Maternal abuse of cocaine, a potent vasoconstrictor, has been associated with fetal stroke. Ischaemic perinatal strokes have been reported in two newborn infants, whose mothers were given prescriptions of codeine-containing cough syrups during pregnancy.[29]

The use of over-the-counter medications and herbal supplements has been on the increase. Dugoua et al.[20] found that 64% of North American midwives had used blue-cohosh, a potent smooth muscle constrictor, as a labour-inducing agent. They reported three infants who had ischaemic perinatal stroke, acute myocardial infarction, and severe multi-organ hypoxic injury, whose mothers had used blue-cohosh during pregnancy.[20]

Neonatal conditions
Both cyanotic and non-cyanotic congenital heart diseases have been associated with systemic venous thrombi and subsequent emboli causing stroke. Infants

Table 4 Clinical features

Neonatal period
- No symptoms: about 30% of infants are discharged as 'normal' during the immediate neonatal period
- Non-specific: lethargy, poor feeding, decreased tone, inactivity, excessive cry
- Seizures
- Encephalopathy with or without coma

Infancy and childhood
- Delayed developmental milestones
- Impaired use of one or more extremities; early 'handedness'
- Clumsy gait, frequent falls
- Unilateral hypo- or hypertonia
- Myoclonic spasms
- Seizures/epilepsy

---

in the intensive care unit in whom in-dwelling vascular catheters have been placed are particularly at higher risk for developing systemic thrombi and emboli.[16,31]

CLINICAL FEATURES

The clinical features of ischaemic perinatal stroke are summarised in Table 4.

Neonatal period
Signs of ischaemic perinatal stroke vary greatly. About one-third of newborns with stroke, as ascertained subsequently, remain asymptomatic with normal neurological examination. They are often sent home as 'normal', only to present with hemiparesis, subtle neurological signs, or seizures later in infancy or childhood.

Seizures are the most common manifestations of ischaemic perinatal stroke to trigger a work-up. Seizures can be unilateral or generalised, and the infant often appears well between the seizures. Some infants with seizures may appear lethargic, progressing into full-fledged signs of encephalopathy. Such infants may be wrongly diagnosed as having 'birth asphyxia' or 'hypoxic-ischaemic encephalopathy'.

Other signs during the neonatal period include sporadic or repeated apnoeas, hypotonia, poor feeding, and irritability. The clinical neurological findings may be normal. It is rare to find unilateral decreased movements or increased neuromuscular tone during the newborn period, even in unilateral ischaemic perinatal stroke.

Infancy and childhood
Infants undiagnosed in the neonatal period may present with seizures during the first year, or later in life. Parents may report delay in achieving developmental milestones, or the child's preference for using one hand more often than the other while reaching for objects beginning at 4–6 months of age when voluntary reaching starts to develop. Such history should trigger a suspicion of developing hemiparesis. The gait may be abnormal or clumsy, with a history of frequent falls. In one study, 70% of infants presented with

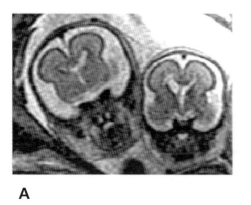
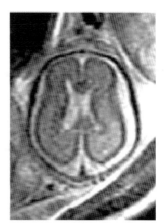

Fig. 1 (A) Axial and (B) coronal fast T2-weighted imaging of twins in utero at approximately 20 weeks' gestational age demonstrating probable subacute ischaemic insult to the parietal region, from twin–twin transfusion syndrome. Note the area of T2 hyperintensity in the parietal region, and some asymmetric effacement of ventricle on the same side. (Images courtesy of Boston Children's Hospital).

seizures, and 30% with a history of early handedness, cerebral palsy or both. Physical examination may reveal findings typical of spastic hemiplegic cerebral palsy.[6,7,15]

RADIOLOGICAL DIAGNOSIS

Fetal stroke

A definitive diagnosis of ischaemic perinatal stroke in the fetus is made using fetal MRI. Brain pathology is first suspected during routine ultrasound studies in normal or in high-risk pregnancies.[19] The ultrasound findings include increased echogenicity from the white matter and a marked asymmetry of the supratentorial ventricular system (Fig. 1A,B).

T2-weighted MRI may reveal hyperintensity, typically in the region of an ischaemic event in the white matter, with or without loss or interruption of the overlying cortical mantle. Diffusion-weighted imaging helps to date the injury and gradient echo imaging helps to identify the presence of altered blood and blood product.

Neonatal stroke

During the neonatal period (especially in sick babies), a bedside cranial ultrasound can be used along with a cerebral Doppler flow study. However, ultrasound studies have limitations. Because of the limited window of the anterior fontanelle, even large lesions can be missed, especially those in the far lateral or posterior brain regions. The quality of an ultrasound study is operator-dependent, and the finding of increased echogenicity is non-specific, since it can occur due to oedema or haemorrhage.

Computed tomography (CT) is the next useful examination (Fig. 2A,B). With advanced, multislice scanners, an unenhanced CT image can be obtained in less than 20 s. CT is excellent for identifying fresh blood and recent haemorrhage; if performed 24 h after an ischaemic event, it may show

115

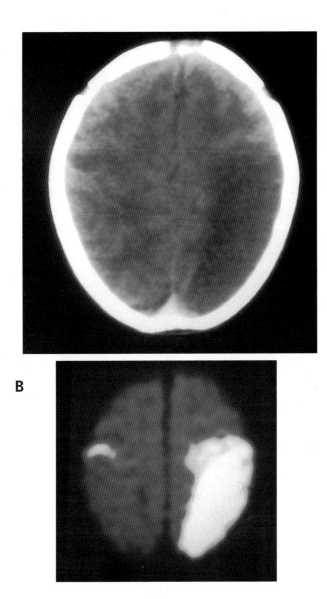

Fig. 2 (A) Axial CT examination on day 2, demonstrating low attenuation returned from the left parietal region with a smaller curvilinear focus of low density in the right parietal region. The presence of more than one ischaemic insult in two different vascular territories suggests the presence of a central embolic source. (B) Axial diffusion-weighted imaging performed on the same day shows restricted diffusion abnormality in the same locations consistent with a recent ischaemic insult.

hypodensity in the area of infarction. In the presence of fresh thrombus, a 'white sign' can be seen outlining the middle cerebral artery. In large vessel infarctions, one can see the classic 'wedge-shaped' areas of low attenuation involving both grey and white matter. Such low density typically fades over 10 days, usually called the 'fogging effect'. CT angiography of the head and neck can be performed using an intravenous bolus of water-soluble iodinated

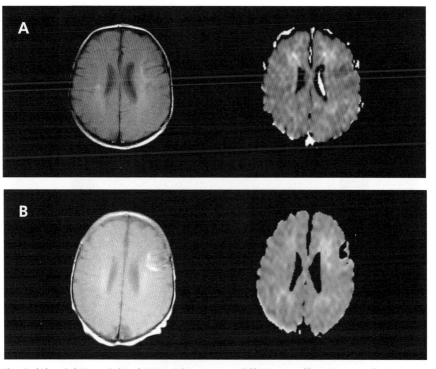

Fig. 3 (A) Axial T1-weighted MRI with apparent diffusion coefficient map of a 9-day-old infant with hypoplastic left heart syndrome. Note the T1 hyperintensity and a matching area of restricted diffusion abnormality in the left frontal region consistent with a recent ischaemic event. (B) Axial T1-weighted MRI with apparent diffusion coefficient map in the same patient, 9 days after surgical correction of hypoplastic left heart syndrome, demonstrating normalisation of apparent diffusion coefficient map, which is the natural history of radiological changes in acute ischaemic events.

contrast material, which outlines the arterial and venous structures, and reveals filling defects or abrupt cut-off of arteries in the presence of distal emboli.

MRI is the most definitive diagnostic examination for ischaemic perinatal stroke (Figs 3–5).[37–40] The examination takes more time than a CT, and may require some sedation. However, by timely feeding and swaddling, and using specially designed padded 'papoose' board (Olympic Medical, Seattle, WA, USA), sedation can be avoided. Ear plugs and muffs must be used to protect hearing.

On T1-weighted imaging (ideally a 3-D volumetric acquisition to obtain thin slices), recent foci of ischaemia will appear hyperintense. On conventional T2-weighted sequences, such areas are correspondingly hypo-intense in the absence of haemorrhage. However, because of the lack of myelination in the newborn period, some signal changes can be difficult to appreciate.

In infarctions of large vessel territories, wedge-shaped areas of abnormality with thinning or loss of the normal overlying cortical ribbon can be seen. Although some reports indicate that it takes 3 weeks for cortical laminar necrosis to become evident, in our experience (JVH), abnormal T1 hyperintensity from the cortex can be seen as early as 16 days following an

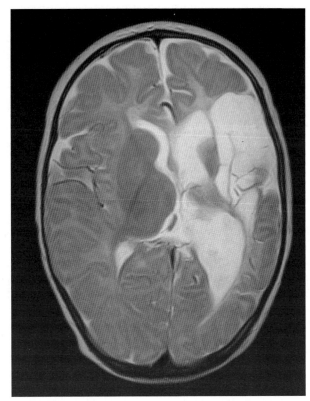

Fig. 4 Presumed perinatal stroke. Axial T2-weighted image in a 6-month-old child with cerebral palsy. Anterior division of left middle cerebral artery shows completed infarction. The child carried the factor V Leiden mutation, possibly causing neonatal arterial infarction.[37]

ischaemic injury. During the acute phase, gadolinium contrast agents are not recommended. After 10 days, these studies can show evidence of blood–brain barrier breakdown.

In diffusion-weighted imaging, the Brownian motion of water in the brain is studied. Following an acute ischaemic insult, the diffusion of water is

Fig. 5 *(opposite page)* (A) Axial unenhanced CT examination of the brain, performed day 13 of life, in an infant with complex congenital heart disease presenting with irritability and seizure. Note bilateral hyperdensities in the region of transverse sinuses, the straight sinus, and the deep internal cerebral veins, suggesting dural venous sinus thrombosis. (B) Sagittal and left parasagittal T1-weighted unenhanced MRI examination of the brain in the same child on day 15 of life demonstrating expansion of and T1 hyperintensity returned from the region of the straight sinus and deep internal cerebral veins, consistent with methaemoglobin and fresh thrombus. Note also, T1 hyperintensity within the left transverse sinus as well as within the white matter paralleling the corpus callosum. (C) Coronal T2-weighted and axial susceptibility-weighted imaging performed same day demonstrating matching T2 hyperintensity returned from the left periventricular white matter, some of which represents haemorrhage (dark on susceptibility-weighted imaging). (D) Coronal and sagittal collapsed maximum intensity projections from a 2-D time-of-flight magnetic resonance venogram, performed without gadolinium administration. Note the absence of flow within the left transverse and sigmoid sinus compared to the right. Note some irregularity and diminution in flow signal returned from the straight sinus and deep internal cerebral veins on the sagittal imaging. The prominent superficial venous drainage overlying the left hemi-cerebrum likely represents evidence for collateral flow, which has opened up to promote venous drainage from the left cerebral hemisphere.

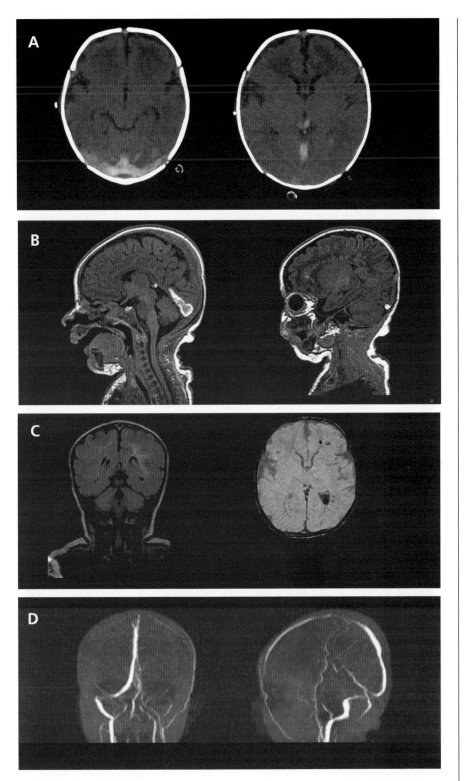

Fig. 5 *(See opposite page for details)*

disturbed. This is reflected as hyperintensity on diffusion data, or hypo-intensity (restriction) on the apparent diffusion coefficient map. This restriction will 'normalise' within 10 days, perhaps as early as 7 days.[37–40] The test takes about 1 min to acquire and post-process.

A 'super' form of diffusion-weighted imaging is diffusion tensor imaging. This takes a longer time to acquire, but can be more informative, since data are collected from 6 or more directions, as compared to 3 for diffusion-weighted imaging. Diffusion tensor imaging allows for measurement of anisotropy, which describes the restriction of the motion of the water constrained by the myelin sheaths that is disturbed or disrupted after an ischaemic event. With diffusion tensor imaging data, robust quantitative analyses can be performed to generate numerical values for apparent diffusion coefficient, fractional anisotropy, primary, secondary and tertiary eigen-vectors to give measures of such parameters as radial diffusivity. These data can also be used to perform 3-D fibre tractography.

Gradient echo imaging can be performed to look for altered blood and blood products. A potentially more sensitive form of gradient echo imaging known as susceptibility-weighted imaging has also been devised to detect tiny amounts of haemorrhage.

Magnetic resonance angiography and venography of the head and neck can be performed using the same instrument to look for evidence of arterial emboli, dissection or stenoses as well as dural venous sinus thrombosis. In general, this is performed without the use of contrast; however, if gadolinium is used, first-pass perfusion data (in a similar way to CT perfusion) can also be acquired to obtain measures of relative cerebral blood flow, relative cerebral blood volume, transit time and time to peak arrival of the bolus of contrast. Mismatches in perfusion/diffusion may have some prognostic value for potential recovery of ischaemic areas as reported in adults.

The 'gold' standard for delineation of arterial and venous anatomy is catheter angiography. However, in contrast to strokes in later childhood, the risk of recurrence of ischaemic perinatal stroke is rare. Therefore, such an invasive procedure may not be indicated.

ANCILLARY STUDIES

Ancillary studies are done to discover the cause of stroke and for counselling. However, there are no uniformly accepted set of investigations to be performed in all cases. One should explore maternal and family history and pregnancy history for risk factors, and consider tests to rule out inherited and acquired prothrombotic and autoimmune conditions listed in Table 2. Even in the presence of thrombotic or autoimmune conditions in the index case (or in the mother), the overall risk of recurrence is about 1.2%, and such strokes seldom occur in other siblings. In patients with Factor V Leiden mutation, the recurrence risk is estimated to be about 3%.

A detailed evaluation is also needed to rule out congenital heart disease and systemic cardiovascular malformations, especially in the region of the neck. An examination of systemic vasculature and of the placenta should be undertaken to find thrombotic lesions.

OUTCOME

Mortality

The mortality rate from ischaemic perinatal stroke is 10% or less in the neonatal period. Mortality rates are higher for fetal strokes. In a review of 118 cases, Ozduman et al.[12] noted that 58 resulted in early fetal deaths, stillbirths or terminations; 14 deaths occurred later in infancy, for a total mortality rate of 61%.

Morbidity

Although many infants with ischaemic perinatal strokes recognised in the newborn period have normal outcome, more than half of infants suffer from varying degrees of neurological and learning disabilities and seizures.[2,4,7,15,16,21–26] The frequency of poor outcomes are: cerebral palsy (78%), cognitive impairment (68%), microcephaly (51%), and seizures (45%). Seizures can be epileptic or infantile spasms; the latter usually precede the former. Neurological disabilities are likely to remain in children in whom ischaemic perinatal stroke is diagnosed retrospectively, after the first few months of life.

The overall IQ can be normal. However, those with repeated seizures and severe MRI abnormalities tend to have lower IQs. Cognitive impairments are more severe in cases with epilepsy. Deficiencies in receptive and expressive language skills are very common, although the effect of age, laterality, and localisation of lesion on language function remains unclear.[41,42] Some, but not all, reports suggest that infants with left hemisphere lesions are worse off in language functions, compared to those with right hemisphere and basal ganglion lesions.

Predictors of poor long-term outcomes

The risks for significant neurological disability are higher with: (i) bilateral ischaemic lesions; (ii) neonatal seizures that are difficult to control; (iii) neonatal EEG with diffuse background abnormalities; (iv) significant neurological abnormality at hospital discharge during the neonatal period; and (v) an early onset of epilepsy.[26]

TREATMENT

Symptomatic therapy

Treatment is directed at alleviating symptoms, and for prevention in those considered to be at-risk for recurrence. Standard antiseizure medications should be prescribed for epilepsy. Other symptomatic therapies include intensive care and ventilatory support as needed.

Thrombolytic therapy

In acute cases, thrombolytic therapy has been recommended, especially if there are thrombi in the heart or the systemic vessels (e.g. catheter-related complications). Anticoagulation therapy may be considered in the presence of one or more plasma-phase risk factors other than factor V Leiden, or the prothrombin gene mutation G2021A, in the presence of a family history of thrombo-embolic events, and when there is radiological confirmation of progression of the lesion.[33]

Evolving therapies

The value of aspirin, heparin, and other thrombolytic agents remains to be studied. Similarly, statins, erythropoeitin, and stem cell therapy are in experimental stages. Mild brain cooling, shown to be beneficial in perinatal encephalopathy, has not been tested in ischaemic perinatal stroke.

SUMMARY

Ischaemic perinatal stroke is emerging as a very important cause of hemiplegic or quadriplegic (total) cerebral palsy, and other long-term neurological disabilities. A high index of suspicion and timely use of advanced neuro-imaging are key to prompt diagnosis. Because of its complex aetiology, obscure presentation, and poor neurological outcome, concerted efforts must be made in the detection, evaluation, and treatment of this condition, preferably using a multidisciplinary team of experts. In a recent publication, Roach et al.[43] provide a comprehensive review of paediatric strokes along with recommendations for their evaluation and management.

Key points for clinical practice

- Suspect perinatal stroke in a newborn infant with persistent, unexplained, non-specific signs and symptoms; and in young infants and children with subtle neurological signs and symptoms, such as developmental delay, clumsy gait, repeated falls, preference for using one upper extremity. Or in any infant or child with seizures, with or without hemiplegia.

- Since the aetiology is multifactorial and possibly cumulative, multiple lines of investigations may be needed to establish the cause of stroke and for counselling purposes; in many cases, precise cause may never be discerned.

- Examination of the placenta and the umbilical cord by an experienced pathologist may be invaluable.

- History to include: prior still births and miscarriages; hypertension; pre-eclampsia; infection; thrombotic conditions; reduced fetal movements; drug abuse; use of prescription medications and over-the-counter herbal preparations; autoantibody screening and fetal ultrasound results; and thrombo-embolic conditions in the family.

- Tests for major thrombotic conditions and autoantibodies can be carried out. Based on the results, screening of siblings and other family members may be considered, especially if multiple systemic sites of thrombosis are found in the index case.

- Cardiovascular system and the neck should be evaluated to rule out structural anomalies and sources of thrombi.

- Magnetic resonance imaging (preferably using advanced techniques) will be the most definitive examination for establishing a diagnosis. Other imaging procedures can also be informative.

(continued)

Key points for clinical practice *(continued)*

- Routine thrombolytic therapy is not recommended. Some infants with acutely progressive cerebral lesions and those with arterial or venous systemic thrombi may benefit from such therapy.

- All patients need to be enrolled into a comprehensive long-term follow-up and rehabilitation programme.

- Besides the paediatrician, other experts may need to be consulted including neurologist, neuroradiologist, haematologist, pathologist (placenta), developmental specialist, and specialist in physical/rehabilitation medicine.

References

1. Wu YW, March WM, Croen LA *et al*. Perinatal stroke in children with motor impairment: a population-based study. *Pediatrics* 2004; **114**: 612–619.
2. Wu YW, Lynch JK, Nelson KB. Perinatal arterial stroke: Understanding mechanisms and outcomes. *Semin Neurol* 2005; **25**: 424–434.
3. Wu, YW, Linda CE, Henning LH *et al*. Neuroimaging abnormalities in infants with congenital hemiparesis. *Pediatr Neurol* 2006; **35**: 191–196.
4. Raju TNK, Nelson KB, Ferriero D, Lynch JK. Ischemic perinatal stroke: Summary of a workshop sponsored by the National Institute of Child Health and Human Development and the National Institute of Neurological Disorders and Stroke. *Pediatrics* 2007; **120**: 609–616.
5. Lsaugesaar R, Kolk A, Tomberg T *et al*. Acutely and retrospectively diagnosed perinatal stroke – a population-based study. *Stroke* 2007; **38**: 2234–2240.
6. Golomb MR, Garg BP, Saha C, Azzouz F, Williams LS. Cerebral palsy after perinatal arterial ischemic stroke. *J Child Neurol* 2008; **23**: 279–286.
7. Golomb MR, Saha C, Garg BP, Azzouz F, Williams LS. Association of cerebral palsy with other disabilities in children with perinatal arterial ischemic stroke. *Pediatr Neurol* 2007; **37**: 245–249.
8. James AH, Bushnell CD, Jamison MG *et al*. Incidence and risk factors for stroke in pregnancy and the puerperium. *Obstet Gynecol* 2005; **106**: 509–516.
9. Benders M, Groenendaal F, Uiterwaal C *et al*. Maternal and infant characteristics associated with perinatal arterial stroke in the preterm infant. *Stroke* 2007; **38**: 1759–1765.
10. Golomb MR, Garg BP, Edwards-Brown M, Williams LS. Very early arterial ischemic stroke in premature infants. *Pediatr Neurol* 2008; **38**: 329–334.
11. Ozduman K, Pober BR, Barnes P *et al*. Fetal stroke. *Pediatr Neurol* 2004; **30**: 151–162.
12. Ozduman K, de Veber G, Ment LR. Stroke in the fetus and the neonate. In: Perlman JM. (ed) *Neurology: Neonatology Questions and Controversies*. Philadelphia, PA: Saunders Elsevier, 2008; 88–121.
13. Fitzgerald KC, Golomb MR. Neonatal arterial ischemic stroke and sinovenous thrombosis associated with meningitis. *J Child Neurol* 2007; **22**: 818–822.
14. Wasay M, Dai AI, Ansari M, Shaikh Z, Roach ES. Cerebral venous sinus thrombosis in children: a multicenter cohort from the United States. *J Child Neurol* 2008; **23**: 26–31.
15. Kirton A, Deveber G, Pontigon AM, Macgregor D, Shroff M. Presumed perinatal ischemic stroke: Vascular classification predicts outcomes. *Ann Neurol* 2008; **63**: 436–443.
16. Beardsley DS. Venous thromboembolism in the neonatal period. *Semin Perinatol* 2007; **3**: 250–253.
17. Schulzke S, Weber P, Leutschg J *et al*. Incidence and diagnosis of unilateral arterial cerebral infarction in newborn infants. *J Perinat Med* 2005; **33**: 170–175.

18. Boffa MC, Lachassinne E. Infant perinatal thrombosis and antiphospholipid antibodies: a review. *Lupus* 2007; **16**: 634–641.

19. Curry CJ, Bhullar S, Holmes J *et al.* Risk factors for perinatal arterial stroke: a study of 60 mother–child pairs. *Pediatr Neurol* 2007; **37**: 99–107.

20. Dugoua J-J, Perri D, Seely D, Mills E, Koren G. Safety and efficacy of blue cohosh (*Caulophyllum thalictroides*) during pregnancy and lactation. *Can J Clin Pharmacol* 2008; **15**: e66–e73.

21. Kenet G, Nowak-Gottl U. Fetal and neonatal thrombophilia. *Obstet Gynecol Clin North Am* 2006; **33**: 457–466

22. Kirton A, deVeber G. Cerebral palsy secondary to perinatal ischemic stroke. *Clin Perinatol* 2006; **33**: 367–386.

23. Kirton A, deVeber G. Perinatal stroke. *Stroke* 2006; **49**: 10–19.

24. Kraus FT, Acheen VI. Fetal thrombotic vasculopathy in the placenta: cerebral thrombi and infarcts, coagulopathies, and cerebral palsy and thrombi in placental vessels of the fetus: insights from litigation. *Hum Pathol* 1999; **30**: 759–769.

25. Lee J, Croen LA, Backstrand KH *et al.* Maternal and infant characteristics associated with perinatal arterial stroke in the infant. *JAMA* 2005; **293**: 723–729.

26. Lee J, Croen LA, Lindan C *et al.* Predictors of outcome in perinatal arterial stroke: a population-based study. *Ann Neurol* 2005; **58**: 303–308.

27. Lo W, Roach ES. The degree of risk: multiple factors promote perinatal stroke. *Pediatr Neurol* 2007; **37**: 152–153.

28. McDonald DGM, Kelehan P, McMenamin JB *et al.* Placental fetal thrombotic vasculopathy is associated with neonatal encephalopathy. *Hum Pathol* 2004; **35**: 875–880.

29. Reynolds EW, Riel-Romero RMS, Bada HS. Neonatal abstinence syndrome and cerebral infarction following maternal codeine use during pregnancy. *Clin Pediatr* 2007; **46**: 639–645.

30. Journeycake JM, Manco-Johnson MJ. Thrombosis during infancy and childhood: what we know and what we do not know. *Hematol Oncol Clin North Am* 2004; **18**: 1315–1338.

31. Hermansen MC, Hermansen MG. Intravascular catheter complications in the neonatal intensive care unit. *Clin Perinatol* 2005; **32**: 141–156.

32. Unal S, Arhan E, Kara N, Uncu N, Aliefendioglu D. Breast-feeding-associated hypernatremia: retrospective analysis of 169 term newborns. *Pediatr Int* 2008; **50**: 29–34.

33. Redline RW, Sagar P, King ME *et al.* Case records of the Massachusetts General Hospital. Case 12-2008. A newborn infant with intermittent apnea and seizures. *N Engl J Med* 2008; **358**: 1713–1723.

34. Jaigobin C, Silver FL. Stroke and pregnancy. *Stroke* 2000; **31**: 2948–2951.

35. Redline RW. Severe fetal placental vascular lesions in term infants with neurologic impairment. *Am J Obstet Gynecol* 2005; **192**: 452–457.

36. Redline RW. Thrombophilia and placental pathology. *Clin Obstet Gynecol* 2006; **49**: 885–894.

37. Thorarenen O, Ryan S, Hunter J, Younkin DP. Factor V Leiden mutation: an unrecognised cause of hemiplegic cerebral palsy, neonatal stroke, and placental thrombosis. *Ann Neurol* 1998; **44**: 426–427.

38. Rutherford M, Counsell S, Allsop J *et al.* Diffusion-weighted magnetic resonance imaging in term perinatal brain injury: a comparison with site of lesion and time from birth. *Pediatrics* 2004; **114**: 1004–1014.

39. Kuker W, Mohrle S, Mader I, Schoning M, Nagele T. MRI for the management of neonatal cerebral infarctions: Importance of timing. *Child Nervous Syst* 2004; **20**: 742–748.

40. Rutherford M, Srinvasan L, Dyet L *et al.* Magnetic resonance imaging in perinatal brain injury: clinical presentation, lesions and outcome. *Pediatr Radiol* 2006; **36**: 582–592.

41. Ricci D, Mercuri E, Barnett A *et al.* Cognitive outcome at early school age in term- born children with perinatally acquired middle cerebral artery territory infarction. *Stroke* 2008; **39**: 403–410.

42. Talib TL, Pongonis SJ, Williams LS *et al.* Neuropsychologic outcomes in a case series of twins discordant for perinatal stroke. *Pediatr Neurol* 2008; **38**: 118–125.

43. Roach ES, Golomb MR, Adams R et al. AHA Scientific Statement. Management of stroke in infants. A scientific statement from a special writing group of the American Heart Association Stroke Council and the Council on Cardiovascular Disease in the Young. *Stroke* 2008; **39**: 2644–2691.

Bahaaldin Alsoufi

New developments in the treatment of hypoplastic left heart syndrome

Hypoplastic left heart syndrome (HLHS) is a term used to describe a heterogeneous group of cardiac malformations characterised by various degrees of underdevelopment of the left heart–aorta complex, resulting in obstruction to systemic cardiac output and the inability of the left heart to support the systemic circulation.[1] Because the neonate with HLHS is dependent on right ventricular ejection through the ductus arteriosus for systemic cardiac output (Fig. 1), continuous infusions of prostaglandins are required to maintain ductal patency. Consequently, surgical stabilisation by any strategy requires revision of the aorta, ductus arteriosus, and pulmonary artery anatomy to achieve the following four objectives: (i) unobstructed systemic cardiac output; (ii) a controlled source of pulmonary blood flow; (iii) a reliable source of coronary blood flow; and (iv) unobstructed egress of pulmonary venous effluent across the atrial septum. The earliest successful palliative first-stage operation was reported by Norwood in 1980 which achieved the treatment objectives described above and has become a mainstay of surgical management for neonates with HLHS.

The natural history of HLHS without surgical intervention is universally fatal. While 'no therapy' has been considered the only appropriate option in the past, this alternative is not commonly offered to otherwise healthy neonates in any advanced congenital cardiac centre due to rapidly improving prognosis recently. Nevertheless, 'no therapy' remains a valid choice in those neonates with severe associated malformations or chromosomal abnormalities that would preclude meaningful survival and quality of life.

The purpose of this review is to evaluate the current results and limitations of several recent developments in the array of currently available management strategies for neonates with HLHS including staged surgical reconstruction, orthotopic heart transplantation, and hybrid palliation.[2–9]

Bahaaldin Alsoufi MD
Consultant in Cardiac Surgery, King Faisal Heart Institute (MBC 16), King Faisal Specialist Hospital and Research Centre, PO Box 3354, Riyadh 11211, Saudi Arabia. E-mail: balsoufi@hotmail.com

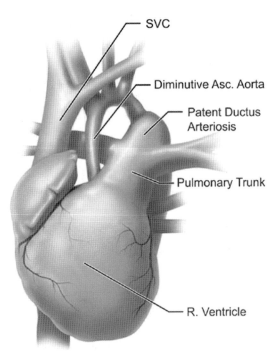

SVC

Diminutive Asc. Aorta

Patent Ductus Arteriosis

Pulmonary Trunk

R. Ventricle

Fig. 1 Anatomical manifestations of HLHS: mitral stenosis or atresia, hypoplasia of the left ventricle, aortic stenosis or atresia, hypoplastic aortic arch, and ductal-dependent systemic cardiac output. Reproduced with permission from *Pediatrics*, vol. **119** (1), pages 109–117, ©2007 by the American Academy of Pediatrics.[42]

STAGED SURGICAL RECONSTRUCTION

OVERVIEW

The Norwood procedure is the most commonly performed initial palliative procedure for patients undergoing staged surgical palliation in the neonatal period.[10] Because the pulmonary vascular resistance is high in the neonatal period, an aortopulmonary shunt or, more recently, a right ventricle to pulmonary artery conduit is used to provide a controlled source of pulmonary blood flow at the cost of volume loading the right ventricle (Fig. 2A,B). A second-stage procedure, the superior bidirectional cavopulmonary anastomosis or hemi-Fontan procedure is typically performed at 4–6 months of age and results in removal of the ventricular volume load by the anastomosis of the superior vena cava to the pulmonary arteries (Fig. 2C). At a third stage, typically at 2–4 years of age, a Fontan procedure is performed to channel the remaining systemic venous return from the inferior vena cava return to the pulmonary arteries (Fig. 2D). Several modifications in operative techniques in each stage have evolved and have contributed to improved surgical results.

THE STANDARD NORWOOD OPERATION UTILISING AN AORTOPULMONARY SHUNT

The standard Norwood procedure utilises an aortopulmonary shunt as the source of pulmonary blood flow (Fig. 3A). Current operative survival in experienced

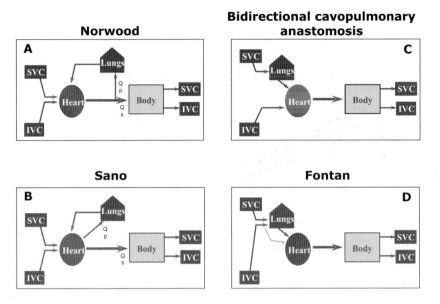

Fig. 2 Schematic representation of the systemic and pulmonary circulation after: (A) Norwood operation with aortopulmonary shunt; (B) Sano modification with right ventricle–pulmonary artery shunt; (C) superior bidirectional cavopulmonary anastomosis; and (D) Fontan procedure. Small arrow in (D) represents a fenestration in the Fontan circuit. SVC, superior vena cava; IVC, inferior vena cava; QS, systemic blood flow; QP, pulmonary blood flow. Reproduced with permission from *Pediatrics*, vol. **119** (1), pages 109–117, ©2007 by the American Academy of Pediatrics.[42]

centres exceeds 70%. Several risk factors for increased operative mortality have been identified such as low birth weight, prematurity, significant associated non-cardiac congenital conditions, delayed presentation, severe pre-operative obstruction to pulmonary venous return, and smaller ascending aorta diameter (Table 1).[1–5,11–13]

Table 1 Surgical outcomes of standard Norwood first stage reconstructive surgery in the treatment of patients with hypoplastic left heart syndrome

Study	Surgery year	No. of patients	Operative mortality	Time-related survival
Bove & Lloyd (1996)[2]	1990–1995	158	24%	5 years, 58%
Daebritz et al. (1999)[3]	1990–1998	131	37%	1 year, 49%
Poirier et al. (2000)[11]	1993–1999	59	17%	1 year, 72%
Mahle et al. (2000)[4]	1984–1999	840	36%	1 year, 51%
				5 years, 40%
				15 years, 39%
Azakie et al. (2001)[5]	1990–2000	171	18%	1 year, 48%
				5 years, 45%
Tweddell et al. (2002)[6]	1992–2001	115	19%	1 year, 66%
				5 years, 61%
Gaynor et al. (2002)[12]	1998–2001	158	22%	1 year, 66%
Ashburn et al. (2003)[13]*	1994–2000	710	28%	1 year, 60%
				5 years, 54%

*Prospective multi-institutional study.

Reproduced with permission from *Pediatrics*, vol. **119** (1), pages 109–117, ©2007 by the American Academy of Pediatrics.[42]

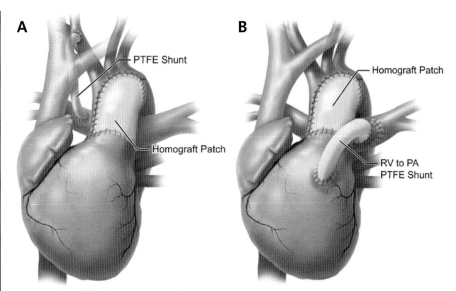

Fig. 3 (A) The final appearance of a completed Norwood operation. The ascending aorta and arch have been reconstructed with homograft patch augmentation. The shunt between the distal innominate artery and the central pulmonary arteries is demonstrated. (B) The final appearance of a completed Sano modification utilising the right ventricle–pulmonary artery shunt. The ascending aorta and arch have been reconstructed with homograft patch augmentation. The shunt between the right ventricle and the central pulmonary arteries including an autologous pericardium cuff is demonstrated.
Reproduced with permission from *Pediatrics*, vol. **119** (1), pages 109–117, © 2007 by the American Academy of Pediatrics.[42]

Achieving consistent early survival following the Norwood procedure remains a major challenge. Because pulmonary blood flow is derived from systemic cardiac output, conventional postoperative management strategies have focused on limitation of pulmonary blood flow by increasing pulmonary vascular resistance using ventilator manipulations with induction of hypoxaemia and hypercarbia. Recently adopted intra-operative and post-operative strategies have included reduction in the size of the aortopulmonary shunt, the use of systemic vasodilators such as phenoxybenzamine, and the continuous monitoring of mixed venous saturation. Using these contemporary measures in the postoperative management following the Norwood operation, some centres were able to achieve hospital survival exceeding 90% in selected groups of patients.[6,7]

Several refinements of operative technique have also been introduced to improve the short- and long-term surgical results. Many studies suggest that prolonged deep hypothermic circulatory arrest is a risk factor for increased operative and inter-stage mortality. Modifications in perfusion management aiming to reduce or eliminate deep hypothermic circulatory arrest by the use of continuous regional cerebral perfusion during arch reconstruction have been adopted by many centres in an effort to decrease operative mortality and the incidence of neurological injury.[14] Although significant advantage has not been collectively demonstrated yet, many surgeons gained increased experience in performing complex arch reconstruction surgery while maintaining continuous selective cerebral perfusion and diminishing or eliminating the duration of brain ischaemia.

Interim mortality remains high and 4–15% of hospital survivors die at home before the second stage operation.[5,12,15] Residual aortic arch obstruction, restrictive atrial septal defects, imbalance of pulmonary and systemic blood flow, diastolic run-off with coronary ischaemia, shunt stenosis or thrombosis, and chronic volume overload of the single ventricle have all been implicated as major causes for inter-stage mortality. In a postmortem study, impairment of coronary perfusion (27%), excessive pulmonary blood flow (19%), obstruction to pulmonary blood flow (17%), neo-aortic obstruction (14%) and right heart failure (13%) were identified as important causes of interim mortality.[16]

Recovery from the critical early postoperative period marks the transition to chronic treatment protocols. While these protocols are different among various centres, they are usually guided by the early postoperative haemodynamics. Most patients are discharged on chronic diuretic therapy with the dose titrated based on clinical findings. Caution is taken to avoid inducing vascular volume depletion with subsequent reduction in cardiac output or hyperviscosity with increased risk for shunt thrombosis. Digoxin is given to patients by some centres, while afterload reduction with an angiotensin converting enzyme inhibitor given selectively to patients with increased Qp/Qs ratio, those who have congestive heart failure, moderate atrioventricular valve insufficiency, or as part of an on-going trial utilising captopril as an afterload reducing agent. For prophylaxis against shunt thrombosis, the protocol varies among centres including antiplatelet therapy with aspirin, Plavix, combination of aspirin and Plavix, or combination along with low molecular weight heparin via subcutaneous injection.

There is a great emphasis on feeding and nutritional support as the infants are commonly incapable of maintaining adequate caloric intake in the early postoperative period. Nutritional requirement in those infants is 100–130 kcal/kg/day. If the patient is unable to take adequate calories with oral feeding alone, a temporary nasogastric feeding tube is initially used and, if necessary, an open gastrostomy tube is placed prior to hospital discharge. It is not recommended to send infants home with nasogastric tubes alone as these can be easily displaced, can interfere with airway protection, increase the incidence of gastro-oesophageal reflux and increase the risk of aspiration. Antireflux medications are often described for patients with evidence of reflux and occasionally antireflux surgery (fundoplication) is required along with the gastrostomy tube insertion.

Finally, aggressive monitoring strategies during this vulnerable period for evidence of cyanosis or overcirculation have resulted in decreased interim mortality.[17] Vigilant postoperative care and monitoring are crucial elements for any successful treatment strategy for HLHS.[17]

Second stage superior bidirectional cavopulmonary anastomosis removes ventricular volume loading and results in a more stable in-series circulation (Fig. 2C). Superior bidirectional cavopulmonary anastomosis is associated with a low operative mortality and subsequent risk of death remains low.[13] The third-stage Fontan procedure (Fig. 2D) is also associated with low operative mortality and a long hazard phase with low mortality.[13]

THE SANO MODIFICATION UTILISING A RIGHT VENTRICLE TO PULMONARY ARTERY SHUNT

The right ventricle–pulmonary artery (RV-PA) shunt to re-establish pulmonary blood supply in stage I palliation for HLHS was first introduced by Norwood in 1981 using large shunts. Due to poor outcomes secondary to excessive pulmonary blood flow and right ventricular failure, the shunt was abandoned in favour of aortopulmonary shunts. Renewed interest in the use of RV-PA shunts has followed increased awareness of its many potential advantages.[18] This modification has been largely popularised by Sano and colleagues[18] and it is called the 'Sano procedure' in many centres (Fig. 3B). Elimination of diastolic run-off into the pulmonary circulation (associated with aortopulmonary shunts) results in higher diastolic pressure and improved coronary perfusion.[19] Additionally, RV-PA shunts are associated with decreased ventricular volume loading and may result in decreased ventricular dilatation, tricuspid valve regurgitation, and reduced interim mortality.[20] Finally, insertion of the RV-PA shunt in the central portion of the pulmonary arteries, provides pulsatile flow that may promote better and more symmetric growth of pulmonary artery.[21]

However, there are some potential disadvantages of the RV-PA shunt. The necessity for a right ventriculotomy may affect the contractile function of the systemic ventricle and may promote ventricular arrhythmias. Moreover, free pulmonary regurgitation of the non-valved conduit may cause ventricular dilatation and contribute to ventricular dysfunction and arrhythmia. RV-PA shunts may be associated with obstruction, occlusion and the development of false aneurysms as well as central pulmonary artery stenosis at the site of shunt

Table 2 Surgical outcomes of the Sano modification first stage reconstructive surgery in the treatment of patients with hypoplastic left heart syndrome utilising right ventricle to pulmonary artery (RV-PA) shunt

Study	Surgery year	Surgery type	Operative mortality	Time-related survival
Mahle et al. (2003)[19]	1999–2002	RV-PA (n = 11)	RV-PA 19%	RV-PA 1 year, 81%
		Norwood (n = 22)	Norwood 19%	Norwood 1 year, 73%
Sano 2004 (18)	1998-2002	RV-PA (n = 73)	16%	1 years 65%
Pizarro et al. (2004)[20]	2000–2003	RV-PA (n = 50) Norwood (n = 46)	RV-PA 8% Norwood 27%	
Bradley et al. (2004)[23]	2000–2003	RV-PA (n = 19) Norwood (n = 25)	RV-PA 11% Norwood 20%	
McGuirk et al. (2005)[22] 50%	1992–2004	RV-PA (n = 73) Norwood (n = 258)	29%	1 year, 58% 10 years,
Tabbutt et al. (2005)[41]	2002–2004	RV-PA (n = 54) Norwood (n = 95)	RV-PA 17% Norwood 14%	

Reproduced with permission from *Pediatrics*, vol. **119** (1), pages 109–117, ©2007 by the American Academy of Pediatrics.[42]

insertion.[21] Lower postoperative oxygen saturations associated with RV-PA shunts may force an early need for the second stage procedure (Table 2).[18–23]

In order to address the knowledge gap in comparing the aortopulmonary and RV-PA shunts, a multicentre, prospective, randomised, clinical trial sponsored by the National Heart, Lung, and Blood Institute is currently underway to evaluate early and intermediate-term outcomes for patients undergoing a Norwood procedure. End-points include death or cardiac transplantation. In addition, the effect of shunt type on intensive care unit morbidity, unintended cardiovascular interventional procedures, right ventricular function, tricuspid valve regurgitation, pulmonary artery growth and neurodevelopmental outcome will be assessed.

Until more data are available to support the benefit of RV-PA shunts, the choice of shunt remains a surgeon's preference. It may have a special role, however, in some high-risk patients such as those with low birth weight, extremely small aorta, pre-operative hypotension, right ventricular dysfunction or tricuspid valve insufficiency, and an aberrant right subclavian artery.

HYBRID STRATEGIES IN THE MANAGEMENT OF HYPOPLASTIC LEFT HEART SYNDROME

Despite major improvements in the outcome of patients following the Norwood procedure, operative and interstage mortality remains substantial. Because the effects of cardiopulmonary bypass and circulatory arrest may contribute to this morbidity and mortality, achieving the critical four objectives enumerated above without utilising cardiopulmonary bypass is potentially an important advance in the management of neonates with HLHS. In addition, suboptimal neurocognitive function among survivors after staged reconstruction has prompted efforts to explore alternatives which avoid cardiopulmonary bypass and circulatory arrest in the neonatal period (Table 3).[24,25]

Ruiz et al.[26] reported experience with stenting of the ductus arteriosus as a bridge to cardiac transplantation in infants with HLHS. Gibbs et al.[27] reported

Table 3 Surgical outcomes of the initial experience with hybrid strategy in the treatment of patients with hypoplastic left heart syndrome

Study	Surgery year	Number	First-stage mortality	Inter-stage mortality	Second-stage mortality	Late death
Akintuerk et al. (2002)[28]	1998–2000	11	0	1/11 (9%)	1/11 (9%)	0
Galantowicz et al. (2005)[29]	2001–2004	29	2/29 (7%)	3/29 (10)%	2/14 (14%)	1/12 (8%)
Pizarro et al. (2005)[30]	2001–2004	10	2/10 (20%)	2/10 (20%)	1/4 (25%)	0
Bacha et al. (2006)[31]	2003–2005	14	3/14 (21%)	2/14 (14%)	2/8 (25%)	1/6 (17%)

the use of a hybrid approach which combined surgery and interventional catheterisation to achieve bilateral pulmonary artery banding, creation of an atrial septal defect and stenting of the arterial duct as an alternative form of

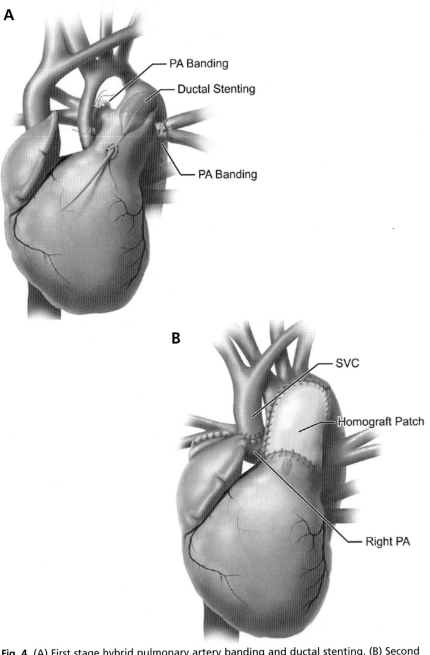

Fig. 4 (A) First stage hybrid pulmonary artery banding and ductal stenting. (B) Second stage reconstruction. The ascending aorta and arch have been reconstructed with homograft patch augmentation. Bidirectional cavopulmonary anastomosis between the superior vena cava and the right pulmonary artery is demonstrated. Reproduced with permission from *Pediatrics*, vol. **119** (1), pages 109–117, ©2007 by the American Academy of Pediatrics.[42]

neonatal palliation for HLHS (Fig. 4A). Multiple authors have subsequently reported small series of neonates undergoing initial palliation with pulmonary artery banding/ductal stenting hybrid procedures with outcomes comparable to current registry data of Norwood procedures.[28–31]

The first-stage pulmonary artery banding/ductal stenting hybrid procedure is typically performed under general anaesthesia in a cardiac catheterisation laboratory equipped to perform surgical procedures with available cardiopulmonary bypass support. The second-stage reconstruction is usually done at 4–6 months of age and consists of stent removal, aortic arch reconstruction and superior bidirectional cavopulmonary anastomosis (Fig. 4B).

Although unproven, the rationale supporting first-stage hybrid palliation with pulmonary artery banding/ductal stenting procedures is predicated on three hypotheses. First, avoidance of cardiopulmonary bypass and cardioplegic arrest as a neonate will result in improved long-term myocardial function. Second, deferring reconstruction of the aortic arch (which requires cardiopulmonary bypass and some alteration in cerebral blood flow and/or circulatory arrest) to an older age (*e.g.* 3–6 months) will result in improved long-term neurological outcomes. And, third, a 3–6-month-old leaving the operating room with an in-series circulation (cavopulmonary shunt) will be more stable than a neonate leaving the operating room with a balanced circulation (aortopulmonary or RV-PA shunt) after a similar operation.

Nonetheless, potential complications of pulmonary artery banding/ductal stenting hybrid procedures include ductal and atrial stent migration, pulmonary artery band migration, stent stenosis and thrombosis.[28–31] Frequent monitoring is needed to detect these complications that may require urgent catheter-based re-interventions or early second-stage reconstruction surgery.[28–31] Immediate or delayed obstruction in the aortic isthmus after stent deployment can become lethal in patients with no prograde aortic flow (*e.g.* aortic atresia) due to acute coronary and cerebral hypoperfusion. In those patients, some have advocated to place a main pulmonary artery to innominate artery graft routinely, which is analogous to a reversed modified Blalock–Taussig shunt, to avoid this problem. Development of intrapulmonary artery flow restrictors, such as the Amplatzer Flow Restrictor, may allow complete stage I palliation in the catheter laboratory without sternotomy.[49]

ORTHOTOPIC HEART TRANSPLANTATION

Since its introduction by Bailey,[32] cardiac transplantation has become a therapeutic alternative for infants with HLHS and remains the preferred treatment in some centres.[33–36] The main advantage of cardiac transplantation is that normal physiology is achieved following a single operation. Although survival following transplantation has been excellent, this approach can not be offered to all infants with HLHS due to limitations in the availability of donor hearts. The overall reported mortality while awaiting transplantation for patients with HLHS is 21–37% (Table 4).[33–38] Furthermore, this approach requires life-long immunosuppression, with the attendant risks of rejection, infection, graft atherosclerosis, and malignancies. While operative mortality is relatively low, survivors continue to experience attrition at a rate of 2% per

Table 4 Surgical outcomes of orthotopic heart transplantation in the treatment of patients with hypoplastic left heart syndrome

Study	Surgery year	Surgery type	Mortality TWL	Oper.	Time-related survival
Razzouk et al. (1996)[33]	1985–95	Transpl. (n = 176)	19%	9%	1 year, 84% 5 years, 76%
Bando et al. (1996)[34]	1989–95	Transpl. (n = 22) Norwood (n = 28)			Transpl. 1 year, 82% Norwood 1 year, 50%
Jenkins * et al. (2000)[38]	1989–94	Transpl. (n = 122)	25%		Transpl. 1 year, 61% Transpl. 5 years, 55%
		Norwood (n = 109)			Norwood 1 year, 42% Norwood 5 years, 38%
Chrisant * et al. (2005)[36]	1993–98	Transpl. (n = 262)	25%	11%	1 year, 92% 5 years, 85%

*Multi-institutional study.
TWL, Transplant waiting list; Oper., Operative
Transpl., Transplantation
Reproduced with permission from *Pediatrics*, vol. **119** (1), pages 109–117, ©2007 by the American Academy of Pediatrics.[42]

year.[35] Survival following transplantation for infants has improved dramatically in the last decade, and future improvements can be expected with the continued advance in the understanding of immune system and the development of new immunosuppressive agents.

One exciting and notable development is the use of ABO-incompatible heart transplantation which exploits the immaturity of the neonatal immune system.[37,39] Newborn infants do not produce isohaemagglutinins and serum anti-A or anti-B antibody titres usually remain low until the age of 12–14 months. Furthermore, the complement system is not fully competent in young infants. Thus, the primary factors that would initiate hyperacute rejection are absent during early infancy.[37,39] This unique immunological opportunity allows the use of ABO-incompatible donor hearts, and can decrease waiting list attrition through expansion of the effective organ donor pool.[37,39]

Another recent development that may increase infant survival while awaiting transplantation is the development of the pulmonary artery banding/ductal stenting hybrid procedures described above. These procedures are equally effective in palliation for neonates awaiting transplantation and allow cessation of prostaglandins, extubation, and discharge home while awaiting a suitable donor. In addition, controlling the pulmonary blood flow may help to minimise the early postoperative pulmonary hypertension, hypoxaemia, and donor right heart failure after transplantation.[28–31] Of note, the use of pulmonary artery banding/ductal stenting pre-transplant hybrid palliation does not preclude 'crossing over' to the staged surgical palliation strategy should a donor heart remain unavailable.

Neonates undergoing transplantation may require subsequent re-transplantation due to the development of allograft vasculopathy and graft dysfunction. Freedom of re-transplantation at 15 years is about 74%.[35,37] Recent reports from experienced centres suggest that survival in children requiring re-transplantation is similar to primary transplantation.[35,40]

Nonetheless, while very few centres offer orthotopic heart transplantation and the primary treatment for neonates with HLHS, staged reconstruction remains the primary procedure offered by most other centres with transplantation performed on those with significant ventricular dysfunction, valvular deformity and regurgitation, or those with a failing heart following first, second or third stage of the reconstruction strategy.[2–9]

SUMMARY

Once considered a uniformly fatal condition, the prognosis of newborns with HLHS has dramatically improved with recent advances in staged reconstructive procedures, pulmonary artery banding/ductal stenting hybrid procedures, and heart transplantation. These techniques are rapidly evolving, and, because individual centres tend to focus on single management strategies with variable reporting of selection and exclusion criteria, it is difficult to compare management strategies across the spectrum of currently available techniques reliably. Multiple multi-institutional studies are currently underway and may help identification of optimum management strategies in this difficult group of patients. In addition, because neonatal survival continues to improve, it is becoming increasingly important to evaluate the long-term consequences of each neonatal management strategy. Life-long follow-up of these children will be needed to allow evaluation of the long-term functional outcomes and health-related quality of life and relate these outcomes to the neonatal choice of management strategy.

Key points for clinical practice

- Hypoplastic left heart syndrome describes a heterogeneous group of cardiac malformations characterised by various degrees of underdevelopment of the left heart–aorta complex, resulting in obstruction to systemic cardiac output and the inability of the left heart to support the systemic circulation.

- Initial management includes prostaglandin infusion to maintain ductal patency and thus systemic perfusion from the right ventricle through the ductus arteriosus.

- Surgical objectives are to provide unobstructed systemic cardiac output, controlled source of pulmonary blood flow, reliable source of coronary blood flow, and unobstructed egress of pulmonary venous effluent across the atrial septum.

- Current surgical options include the Norwood operation, Sano modification, heart transplantation, hybrid palliation and no therapy.

- As surgical outcomes have improved, 'no therapy' is currently offered mainly to neonates with severe associated malformations or chromosomal abnormalities that would preclude meaningful survival and quality of life.

(cont'd)

Key points for clinical practice (cont'd)

- Most mortality in multistage palliation surgery take place following first-stage operation for hypoplastic left heart syndrome in addition to interim mortality before stage-two operation.

- Modifications in operative strategy and intensive care have reduced peri-operative mortality following stage-one palliation in some centres to as low as 10%.

- Discharge medications include furosemide, sometimes digoxin and captopril, aspirin with or without heparin, in addition to special attention to adequate nutrition and prevention of reflux and aspiration.

- Complications related to the aortopulmonary shunt (such as coronary steal, excessive pulmonary flow with low systemic perfusion, and shunt thrombosis) account for the majority of causes of early and interim deaths following the standard Norwood procedure.

- Home monitoring adopted by some programmes has proved helpful detecting early anatomical and haemodynamic problems and decreasing interim mortality.

- There has been recent enthusiasm to adopting the right ventricle–pulmonary artery modification of the Norwood operation (Sano procedure) to avoid shunt-related complications.

- Potential right ventricle–pulmonary artery conduit advantages include elimination of coronary steal, improved systemic perfusion, decreased volume load, and improved pulmonary artery growth.

- Potential right ventricle–pulmonary artery conduit disadvantages include ventricular arrhythmias and dysfunction, free pulmonary regurgitation through the conduit, conduit narrowing and lower oxygen saturations necessitating early, second-stage operation.

- Results of many institutional series vary and a prospective multicentre US National Institutes of Health trial is underway to determine advantage of right ventricle–pulmonary artery modification over standard Norwood with aortopulmonary shunt.

- There is evidence of suboptimal neurocognitive function among survivors after staged reconstruction for hypoplastic left heart syndrome. This may be due to exposure to prolonged cardio-pulmonary bypass and circulatory arrest in the neonatal period.

- Hybrid procedures with ductal stenting, atrial septostomy and pulmonary artery banding were adopted recently to avoid prolonged bypass and circulatory arrest in the neonatal period.

- Hybrid procedure results are encouraging although complications have been frequently reported mainly due to learning curve. Recent reports showed a decrease in those technical problems.

(cont'd)

Key points for clinical practice *(cont'd)*

- Operative mortality for second-stage palliation (Glenn versus hemi-Fontan) and third-stage palliation (Fontan) have significantly decreased and several operative modifications have been developed.

- Heart transplantation allows the infant to have normal cardiac physiology following a single operation and has been adopted by some centres as the treatment of choice.

- Problems with transplantation include high pre-transplant mortality while waiting for appropriate donor, in addition to problems related to life-long immunosuppression, with the attendant risks of rejection, infection, graft atherosclerosis, and malignancies.

- While re-transplantation survival has improved, staged reconstruction remains the primary procedure offered by most centres with transplantation performed on those with significant ventricular dysfunction, valvular deformity and regurgitation, or those with a failing heart following first, second or third stage of the reconstruction strategy.

- Surgical strategies are rapidly evolving and further follow-up is necessary to determine optimal treatment choice.

- As survival continues to improve, it is becoming increasingly important to evaluate the long-term consequences of each neonatal management strategy and to evaluate long-term functional outcomes and health-related quality of life and relate these outcomes to the neonatal choice of management strategy.

References

1. Tchervenkov CI, Jacobs ML, Tahta SA. Congenital Heart Surgery Nomenclature and Database Project: hypoplastic left heart syndrome. *Ann Thorac Surg* 2000; **69 (Suppl)**: S170–S179.
2. Bove EL, Lloyd TR. Staged reconstruction for hypoplastic left heart syndrome. Contemporary results. *Ann Surg* 1996; **224**: 387–394.
3. Daebritz SH, Nollert GD, Zurakowski D *et al*. Results of Norwood stage I operation: comparison of hypoplastic left heart syndrome with other malformations. *J Thorac Cardiovasc Surg* 2000; **119**: 358–367.
4. Mahle WT, Spray TL, Wernovsky G, Gaynor JW, Clark 3rd BJ. Survival after reconstructive surgery for hypoplastic left heart syndrome: a 15-year experience from a single institution. *Circulation* 2000; **102 (Suppl 3)**: III136–III141.
5. Azakie T, Merklinger SL, McCrindle BW *et al*. Evolving strategies and improving outcomes of the modified Norwood procedure: a 10-year single-institution experience. *Ann Thorac Surg* 2001; **72**: 1349–1353.
6. Tweddell JS, Hoffman GM, Mussatto KA *et al*. Improved survival of patients undergoing palliation of hypoplastic left heart syndrome: lessons learned from 115 consecutive patients. *Circulation* 2002; **106 (Suppl 1)**: I82–I89.
7. Bradley SM, Atz AM. Postoperative management: the role of mixed venous oxygen saturation monitoring. *Semin Thorac Cardiovasc Surg Pediatr Card Surg Annu* 2005; **8**: 22–27.

8. Razzouk AJ, Chinnock RE, Gundry SR *et al.* Transplantation as a primary treatment for hypoplastic left heart syndrome: intermediate-term results. *Ann Thorac Surg* 1996; **62**: 1–7.

9. Chrisant MR, Naftel DC, Drummond-Webb J *et al.* Fate of infants with hypoplastic left heart syndrome listed for cardiac transplantation: a multicenter study. *J Heart Lung Transplant* 2005; **24**: 576–582.

10. Norwood WI, Kirklin JK, Sanders SP. Hypoplastic left heart syndrome: experience with palliative surgery. *Am J Cardiol* 1980; **45**: 87–91.

11. Poirier NC, Drummond-Webb JJ, Hisamochi K *et al.* Modified Norwood procedure with a high-flow cardiopulmonary bypass strategy results in low mortality without late arch obstruction. *J Thorac Cardiovasc Surg* 2000; **120**: 875–884.

12. Gaynor JW, Mahle WT, Cohen MI *et al.* Risk factors for mortality after the Norwood procedure. *Eur J Cardiothorac Surg* 2002; **22**: 82–89.

13. Ashburn DA, Blackstone EH, Wells WJ *et al.* Determinants of mortality and type of repair in neonates with pulmonary atresia and intact ventricular septum. *J Thorac Cardiovasc Surg* 2004; **127**: 1000–1007.

14. Pigula FA. Arch reconstruction without circulatory arrest: scientific basis for continued use and application to patients with arch anomalies. *Semin Thorac Cardiovasc Surg Pediatr Card Surg Annu* 2002; **5**: 104–115.

15. Mahle WT, Spray TL, Gaynor JW, Clark 3rd BJ. Unexpected death after reconstructive surgery for hypoplastic left heart syndrome. *Ann Thorac Surg* 2001; **71**: 61–65.

16. Bartram U, Grunenfelder J, Van Praagh R. Causes of death after the modified Norwood procedure: a study of 122 postmortem cases. *Ann Thorac Surg* 1997; **64**: 1795–1802.

17. Ghanayem NS, Cava JR, Jaquiss RD, Tweddell JS. Home monitoring of infants after stage one palliation for hypoplastic left heart syndrome. *Semin Thorac Cardiovasc Surg Pediatr Card Surg Annu* 2004; **7**: 32–38.

18. Sano S, Ishino K, Kawada M, Honjo O. Right ventricle-pulmonary artery shunt in first-stage palliation of hypoplastic left heart syndrome. *Semin Thorac Cardiovasc Surg Pediatr Card Surg Annu* 2004; **7**: 22–31.

19. Mahle WT, Cuadrado AR, Tam VK. Early experience with a modified Norwood procedure using right ventricle to pulmonary artery conduit. *Ann Thorac Surg* 2003; **76**: 1084–1088.

20. Pizarro C, Mroczek T, Malec E, Norwood WI. Right ventricle to pulmonary artery conduit reduces interim mortality after stage 1 Norwood for hypoplastic left heart syndrome. *Ann Thorac Surg* 2004; **78**: 1959–1963.

21. Rumball EM, McGuirk SP, Stumper O *et al.* The RV-PA conduit stimulates better growth of the pulmonary arteries in hypoplastic left heart syndrome. *Eur J Cardiothorac Surg* 2005; **27**: 801–806.

22. McGuirk SP, Griselli M, Stumper O *et al.* Staged surgical management of hypoplastic left heart syndrome: a single-institution 12-year experience. *Heart* 2006; **92**: 364–370.

23. Bradley SM, Simsic JM, McQuinn TC *et al.* Hemodynamic status after the Norwood procedure: a comparison of right ventricle-to-pulmonary artery connection versus modified Blalock–Taussig shunt. *Ann Thorac Surg* 2004; **78**: 933–941.

24. Mahle WT, Wernovsky G. Neurodevelopmental outcomes in hypoplastic left heart syndrome. *Semin Thorac Cardiovasc Surg Pediatr Card Surg Annu* 2004; **7**: 39–47.

25. Galli KK, Zimmerman RA, Jarvik GP *et al.* Periventricular leukomalacia is common after neonatal cardiac surgery. *J Thorac Cardiovasc Surg* 2004; **127**: 692–704.

26. Ruiz CE, Gamra H, Zhang HP, Garcia EJ, Boucek MM. Stenting of the ductus arteriosus as a bridge to cardiac transplantation in infants with the hypoplastic left-heart syndrome. *N Engl J Med* 1993; **328**: 1605–1608.

27. Gibbs JL, Wren C, Watterson KG, Hunter S, Hamilton JR. Stenting of the arterial duct combined with banding of the pulmonary arteries and atrial septectomy or septostomy: a new approach to palliation for the hypoplastic left heart syndrome. *Br Heart J* 1993; **69**: 551–555.

28. Akintuerk H, Michel-Behnke I, Valeske K *et al.* Stenting of the arterial duct and banding of the pulmonary arteries: basis for combined Norwood stage I and II repair in hypoplastic left heart. *Circulation* 2002; **105**: 1099–1103.

29. Galantowicz M, Cheatham JP. Lessons learned from the development of a new hybrid strategy for the management of hypoplastic left heart syndrome. *Pediatr Cardiol* 2005; **26**: 190–199.

30. Pizarro C, Murdison KA. Off pump palliation for hypoplastic left heart syndrome: surgical approach. *Semin Thorac Cardiovasc Surg Pediatr Card Surg Annu* 2005; **8**: 66–71.

31. Bacha EA, Daves S, Hardin J *et al*. Single-ventricle palliation for high-risk neonates: The emergence of an alternative hybrid stage I strategy. *J Thorac Cardiovasc Surg* 2006; **131**: 163–171.

32. Bailey LL. Role of cardiac replacement in the neonate. *J Heart Transplant* 1985; **4**: 506–509.

33. Razzouk AJ, Chinnock RE, Gundry SR *et al*. Transplantation as a primary treatment for hypoplastic left heart syndrome: intermediate-term results. *Ann Thorac Surg* 1996; **62**: 1–7.

34. Bando K, Turrentine MW, Sun K *et al*. Surgical management of hypoplastic left heart syndrome. *Ann Thorac Surg* 1996; **62**: 70–76.

35. Bailey LL. Transplantation is the best treatment for hypoplastic left heart syndrome. *Cardiol Young* 2004; **14 (Suppl 1)**: 109–111.

36. Chrisant MR, Naftel DC, Drummond-Webb J *et al*. Fate of infants with hypoplastic left heart syndrome listed for cardiac transplantation: a multicenter study. *J Heart Lung Transplant* 2005; **24**: 576–582.

37. Boucek Jr RJ, Chrisant MR. Cardiac transplantation for hypoplastic left heart syndrome. *Cardiol Young* 2004; **14 (Suppl 1)**: 83–87.

38. Jenkins PC, Flanagan MF, Jenkins KJ *et al*. Survival analysis and risk factors for mortality in transplantation and staged surgery for hypoplastic left heart syndrome. *J Am Coll Cardiol* 2000; **36**: 1178–1185.

39. West LJ, Pollock-Barziv SM, Dipchand AI *et al*. ABO-incompatible heart transplantation in infants. *N Engl J Med* 2001; **344**: 793–800.

40. Dearani JA, Razzouk AJ, Gundry SR *et al*. Pediatric cardiac retransplantation: intermediate-term results. *Ann Thorac Surg* 2001; **71**: 66–70.

41. Tabbutt S, Dominguez TE, Ravishankar C *et al*. Outcomes after the stage I reconstruction comparing the right ventricular to pulmonary artery conduit with the modified Blalock Taussig shunt. *Ann Thorac Surg* 2005; **80**: 1582–1590.

42. Alsoufi B, Bennets J, Verma S, Caldarone CA. New developments in the treatment of hypoplastic left heart syndrome. *Pediatrics* 2007; **119**: 109–117.

Elizabeth A. Mitchell R. Scott Dingeman

10

Parent presence during cardiopulmonary resuscitation and complex invasive procedures

INTRODUCTION

HISTORICAL CONTEXT

The concept of offering parents the option to be present while complex invasive procedures are being performed on their child and/or during cardiopulmonary resuscitation (CPR) is a relatively new and controversial practice, which has elicited emotional responses from both parents and clinicians alike. Family-member presence during adult resuscitations, on the other hand, has received nation-wide attention since the 1980s when clinicians at the Emergency Department of the W.A. Foote Memorial Hospital in Jackson, Michigan first reported their experience with family-member presence during resuscitations. In their ground-breaking study, these researchers found that 72% of family members who lost a loved one during cardiac arrest wished they had been present during the resuscitation attempt. Furthermore, no family-member interference occurred during the study period.[1] Based on these findings, a protocol allowing selective family-member presence was implemented in the adult care-units. Before long, other hospitals conducted studies and some implemented policies for the practice of family presence during invasive procedures and cardiopulmonary resuscitation. Paediatric research has been slower to evolve in this area, but the breadth of literature is fast-growing. There is now over a decade of studies from both the US and the UK

Elizabeth A. Mitchell BS
Research Project Co-ordinator, Cardiovascular and Critical Care Programs, Children's Hospital
Boston, 300 Longwood Avenue, Farley 603, Boston, MA 02114, USA
E-mail: elizabeth.mitchell@childrens.harvard.edu

R. Scott Dingeman MD FAAP (for correspondence)
Instructor of Anaesthesia, Harvard Medical School and Assistant in Peri-operative Anesthesia and
Pain Medicine, Children's Hospital Boston, 300 Longwood Avenue, Boston, MA 02118, USA
E-mail: scott.dingeman@childrens.harvard.edu

emphasising the benefits of the parent component in the parent–child–clinician dynamic, and this research has been contributing to the evolving phenomenon of family-centred care within paediatric hospitals.

FAMILY-CENTRED CARE AND ITS IMPACT ON THE PRACTICE OF PARENT PRESENCE

Paediatric patients are unique to medicine since a parent or guardian who often accompanies them not only makes medical decisions on their behalf, but is also their primary source of support attending to their daily emotional, social, and physical needs. The philosophy of family-centred care emphasises the importance of meeting not only the physical needs of children but also their psychosocial and developmental needs; therefore, it encourages clinicians to recognise the major impact families may have on the health and well-being of their children. It is now well-accepted that paediatric care should be provided within the context of families. In many out-patient and hospital settings, parents and guardians are commonly present during some of their child's invasive procedures, such as the insertion of peripheral intravenous or Foley catheters or during lumbar puncture. At some institutions, parents are present during the induction of elective anaesthesia for invasive procedures or surgery. Thus, one of the last bastions of this evolving phenomenon is re-thinking the practice of routinely asking parents to leave the bedside during more invasive procedures in acute-care settings, such as central venous cannulation, chest tube insertion, endotracheal intubation, and/or cardiopulmonary resuscitation.

PARENT PRESENCE DURING COMPLEX INVASIVE PROCEDURES AND CARDIOPULMONARY RESUSCITATION

Few institutions routinely offer parents the option to remain with their child during complex invasive procedures and/or CPR, and even fewer have guidelines or policies to help facilitate this process. The literature reveals that apprehensions and controversy abound among clinicians regarding parent presence and opinions vary widely regarding the appropriateness and logistical feasibility of the practice. Given the lack of clinician consensus, there is wide unit-to-unit and clinician-to-clinician variation regarding parent presence. Parents, on the other hand, clearly prefer to have the choice about whether or not they remain at their child's bedside during these events. In 2000, the American Heart Association was the first national organisation to endorse a guideline that recommended that parents be given the option to be present during their child's invasive procedure and/or resuscitation.[2–8] Since that time, several other national organisations within the US, including the American Academy of Pediatrics, the American College of Emergency Physicians, and the Society of Critical Care Medicine have lent their endorsement to the practice of parent presence. These recommendations, in concert with growing public awareness,[9–11] are compelling and are prompting more discussion by paediatric facilities about the need to re-examine their practices and to develop formal institutional guidelines for parent presence during highly invasive procedures and CPR. In 2003, the National Consensus

Conference on Family Presence during Pediatric Cardiopulmonary Resuscitation and Procedures convened clinicians from 18 national organisations to develop guidelines that may be useful in defining an institutional policy for the practice of parent presence.[12] The recommendations have laid a foundation for paediatric hospitals to advance their practices around ensuring comprehensive and effective family-centre care.

IMPLICATIONS FOR PAEDIATRIC CLINICIANS

This chapter presents a comprehensive review of the literature on parental presence during both complex invasive procedures and CPR. The research-based directives can help guide clinicians to make informed decisions when offering parents the option to stay during these potentially complicated events.

CURRENT PRACTICE

Clinicians are most concerned about the possibility that parents who remain present during complex invasive procedures and/or CPR will interfere with, or obstruct, patient care. These concerns and fears on the part of clinicians are largely unfounded in the literature. However, these underlying worries serve to fuel ambivalence, reluctance, and lack of support for parent presence. The literature suggests a growing trend that, when given the option, more parents are choosing to stay with their child during an invasive procedure and/or resuscitation, and those who have done so would repeat their choice in the future.[9,13,14] Despite the expressed wishes of parents to have a choice, research studies have found that parents are not routinely being offered the option to stay.[13,15–18] In the up-dated American Heart Association Emergency and Critical Care and CPR guidelines, the statement was made that: 'Parents or family members seldom ask if they can be present unless they have been encouraged to do so. Healthcare providers should offer the opportunity to family members whenever possible.' Such advice is telling.

In 1991, Bauchner et al.[13] reported that less than half of parents surveyed would want to be present if their child was undergoing an invasive procedure in the emergency department. Almost a decade later, Boie et al.[9] reported that 87% of the parents they surveyed would want to be present if their child was undergoing an invasive procedure and 83% of parents would want to be present during resuscitation events. In 2006, Gold et al.[20] reported that of the paediatric/neonatal intensive care unit and paediatric/general emergency resuscitation physician sample surveyed, 68% reported that most parents wanted the option to be present. In 2005, the majority of parents surveyed in the emergency department said that they not only wanted to be present, but also 86% believed it was their right to be present.[21] Conclusions by Boie and colleagues[9] are consistent with these findings and suggest that parents wish to have a choice about being present at the bedside, and they do not want clinicians to decide on their behalf whether they should stay or leave their child's beside. In the Sacchetti et al.[22] study, of the six parents who felt that parent presence was a bad idea, five stood at the beside while one helped restrain the child; four of the six felt their presence helped their child and would remain again.

In retrospect, after experiencing their child's invasive procedure or resuscitation, most parents do not regret their decision to be present. In a US paediatric intensive care unit, Powers et al.[14] reported that 94% of parents given the option to be present would repeat their decision to stay. Similarly, in the emergency department setting, Mangurten et al.[21] reported that all parents agreed or strongly agreed that they would repeat their decision to remain at their child's bedside. No research to date has investigated the potential for parents to develop serious symptoms of post-traumatic stress syndrome from witnessing CPR on their child.

The literature suggests that parental decision-making to remain present is not related to parental age, gender, race, marital status, level of education,[9,13] or income.[9] In the emergency department, Bauchner and colleagues[13] found that a parent's previous experience with a procedure and/or resuscitation increased the likelihood that the parent would choose to stay again. Severity of the child's condition influenced the parental desire to be present, with 71% wanting to be present if their child was unconscious and 83% if death were likely.[9] Additionally, 81% of the parents said they would want to be present when their child was conscious.

Clinician support for parent presence during invasive procedures and resuscitation appears to vary by discipline, geographical region, and hospital department. Nurses are more likely to consent to parent presence during invasive procedures[21,23] and resuscitation[16,17,21] than attending physicians[16,17] or physicians-in-training.[21,23,24] Fein and colleagues[25] found that attending physicians and nurses were significantly more likely than physicians-in-training to approve or consider family member presence during both invasive procedures and resuscitation efforts. Clinicians from in-patient settings were more willing to permit parent presence during resuscitation compared to those from out-patient settings ($P < 0.001$).[24] A single study found that physicians with additional training in emergency medicine and paediatric emergency medicine had a higher level of comfort and were much more likely to encourage parents to stay during procedures than were general paediatricians.[18] In contrast, the most recent report by Gold et al.,[20] examining physicians from different geographic, institutional and specialty areas, reported that a favourable opinion of family presence did not differ by provider gender, age, parental status (i.e. being a parent or not), being a paediatric provider, or having a personal history of witnessing cardiopulmonary resuscitation on a family member. For the clinician who opposed family presence, the majority wrote comments that they believed being present during resuscitation would be haunting and traumatic for families. Interestingly, the study of physicians in UK by Booth et al.[15] found that, regardless of policies/guidelines of their own departments, 85% of physicians said they would prefer to be present during resuscitation if it was their own child.

Clinicians are more likely to support parent presence during less invasive procedures[13,18,21,25] and when patients did not have life-threatening conditions.[18,25] Several of the studies corroborated findings that the more invasive the procedure, the less likely clinicians were to offer parents the option to remain.[13,18,21,25] Study findings asking clinicians whether they would honour a parent's request to remain during their child's resuscitation varied widely, from 22% to 93%.[15,16,18,20,24] Of clinicians, 39–90% either agreed that they would continue the practice of allowing parents to be present or that they would continue to give parents the option to be present in future procedures and/or resuscitations.[16,18,21,23,24] An evaluation of the literature over time shows that the level of physician support for family presence has become markedly higher. Both the expansion of family-centred care and the implementation of hospital policies on the practice of parent presence have likely caused this increase in acceptance.

COMMON BEDSIDE BEHAVIOUR BY PARENTS

Parents have become increasingly more active participants in their child's healthcare. Sacchetti and colleagues conducted two studies in a university-affiliated emergency department and noted that parent activity during invasive procedures was self-initiated with parents typically standing at the bedside.[23,26] Less invasive procedures were observed in the earlier 1996 study, and it was found that 50% of parents helped in restraining the child and other activities such as providing soothing attention.[23] In 2006, Mangurten and colleagues[21] reported that all parents emotionally supported their child, most (91%) talked to and/or soothed their child, and 73% touched and/or kissed their child. Half the parents functioned as an additional and/or familiar set of hands, to help settle and restrain patients when necessary during invasive procedures.[21] Studies regarding the inclusion of parents during induction of anaesthesia have found that parent involvement decreased parental stress and allowed them to be a trusted presence in the room for their child.

The paediatric literature provides evidence that parents did not generally interfere with their child's care during invasive procedures or resuscitation, and serious parental interference was not reported during any of the studies. In fact, all studies in which parent behaviour was reported, parent interferences were minimal and almost all easily addressed. In one of six surveys examining parental interference with patient care,[14,15,21,23,26,27] Sacchetti et al.[26] reported some minor interference that did not alter patient care. In the only Randomised Control Trial (RCT), parents did not interrupt the resuscitation or delay the decision to discontinue resuscitation efforts.[27] No parent was asked to leave nor did parents report being frightened by the process. Mangurten et al.[21] reported that over 90% of clinicians felt the family's behaviour had not been disruptive to patient care and that the treatments given were the same, with procedures requiring approximately the same length of time. Almost 90% of clinicians said their procedural performance was not affected by parental presence. Similarly, family presence did not interfere with medical student or resident training in two emergency department studies.[21,23] In 2005, 71% of clinicians (mostly physicians) with membership of the American Academy of Pediatrics and the American College of Emergency Physicians reported that family-member presence was allowed in their institution if residents were participating in CPR, although three-quarters felt that it could intimidate residents. In addition, 79% felt that paediatric residents should receive training in family presence during CPR.[20] Informed parents are calmer parents, and it is the recommendation of these authors that clinicians receive preparation techniques teaching about the need to inform the parents of their options, give procedural steps and time-frames, explain potential procedure outcomes, and let the parents know they will be supported throughout their experience whether they choose to stay or remain in the room.

BENEFITS AND RISKS

As a result of family-centred care initiatives, parents or guardians are now being offered the option to remain present during complex invasive procedures and/or during CPR with several favourable benefits to both the child and the parent or guardian. Potential benefits to the child include the availability of the parent or guardian to calm an anxious or unco-operative child and to participate and assist in the care of their child directly.[13,14,21,23,25,26] Potential benefits to parents themselves include decreased parental anxiety and feelings of helplessness, increased parental knowledge of their child's illness and treatments, acceptance by parents that everything was done for their child, and facilitation of the grieving process for the bereaved parent.[14,16,23,25,27] Study results have also found that clinicians gain advantages from the presence of parents. Under the best of circumstances, parent presence offers an opportunity to build rapport with the clinicians caring for their child during these significant events.[16,21,25] Some clinicians suggest that parent presence may actually reduce suspicions by the parents and, therefore, decrease the risk of litigation.[16] However, there appears to be no consensus in the literature among clinicians as to the potential benefits that parents may have on the healthcare team during these situations.[18,21,25]

PATIENT PERSPECTIVES

Paediatric patients are unique since parents and guardians who often accompany them not only make medical decisions on their behalf, but also serve as their primary source of support by attending to their daily emotional, social, and physical needs. Yet the value of parent presence on paediatric patients has not been well studied or addressed with direct measurement of child discomfort, ease, personal preference, or sense of humanity. Although comparable data do not exist in children, Robinson et al.[27] reported that adult resuscitation survivors did not believe their confidentiality or dignity was compromised by family-member presence. These adult patients also expressed that their family members' presence made them feel less alone and that they were content that the family member was present.[27] The clinicians in the initial study conducted by Sacchetti et al.[23] speculated that, when a parent is not present, a child may be more likely to internalise feelings; however, they did not study or comment upon whether they thought this would be beneficial or harmful.

Medical literature indicates there is increased clinician anxiety related to fear of a parent's lack of ability to support his or her child during painful and serious procedures. Still, the majority of parents, both those who had been present and those who had not, would opt to accompany their child during procedures and resuscitation. Eichhorn et al.[28] reported some of the benefits described by several adolescent and adult patients undergoing invasive procedures and one surviving patient who underwent resuscitation. These patients described the presence of their family member or spouse as comforting and beneficial in providing help and reminding providers of their personhood. In addition, these patients believed that the benefits to their family members outweighed the potential problems, and none of these patients reported feeling embarrassed or undignified due to the presence of a family member or spouse.[28] Given the nature of the parent–child relationship, the influence of parent presence on infants and younger children is an area ripe for further study.

PARENTAL PERSPECTIVES

Most parents believed that their presence during invasive procedures and resuscitations helped their child[14,21,23] or helped them.[13,14,21,23] Parents agreed or strongly agreed that being able to be present provided them with peace of mind, allowed them to let their child know they loved them, and helped them know that everything possible had been done to treat their child.[21] On standardised questionnaires, Robinson et al.[27] found positive trends in the psychological health of family members, such that family members who remained present during resuscitations had lower anxiety and depression scores, fewer disturbing memories, and lower degrees of intrusive imagery and post-traumatic avoidance behaviour 3 months after the event. This particular study was terminated early because clinicians became convinced that family presence was beneficial for relatives. Similarly, Mangurten and colleagues[21] reported that most parents felt being present helped ease their grief. In the paediatric intensive care setting, Powers et al.[14] reported that parents who were given the option to accompany their child at the bedside had significantly less anxiety related to the procedure than the control group who were not allowed to be present ($P = 0.005$). In a tertiary care emergency department, Fein and colleagues[25] documented the advantages of family-member presence to be decreased fears of the unknown and feelings of helplessness and/or increased feelings of usefulness.

CLINICIAN PERSPECTIVES

From the literature, it is clear that offering parents the option to remain at the bedside during their child's invasive procedure and/or resuscitation is a controversial practice. Much of the controversy arises because clinicians differ in their opinion as to what might be the best for the child and for the parent. Yet since the pioneering studies of the Foote Hospital, research has consistently shown that providing the option for families to be present not only benefits families, but also clinicians. Several studies have suggested that parental presence might be beneficial to clinicians during invasive procedures and resuscitations.[18,21,25] Specifically, clinicians in the Fein et al.[25] study felt parent presence facilitated parent education, forged rapport, and enabled parents to help the medical team during the procedure. Jarvis et al.[16] found that 62% of paediatric intensive care unit physicians believed if a child were to die, family member bereavement would be helped if they had witnessed CPR. Of clinicians who had experience with family presence during paediatric resuscitations, 65% felt it was more helpful to families when the child died versus 53% when the child survived, and 61% felt it was more helpful to families with a child that had a chronic medical condition versus 51% for a previously well child.[20]

Four studies have reported that parent presence might be detrimental to clinicians and their performance during resuscitation, with 22–85% not in favour of the practice,[17,18,24,25] and three studies which also included invasive procedures reported clinicians to have unfavourable attitudes towards the practice.[18,22,25] Physicians said they opposed family presence during resuscitation because it engendered performance anxiety and medicolegal concerns.[15,17,21,25] Other clinicians, however, believed that parent presence might actually reduce suspicions and the risk of litigation because it might help parents gain a realistic view of the attempted resuscitation.[16] A quarter of clinicians in the Mangurten et al.[21] study were concerned that a parent might misinterpret treatment activities. Other disadvantages that were mentioned included a change in interpersonal dynamics,[21] the need for additional staff resources or time,[25] and increased nervousness/stress of staff.[13,16,18,20] Jarvis[16] reported that clinicians in the UK felt family presence during resuscitations might inhibit treatment by junior staff, and clinicians at a children's hospital reported that it might compromise teaching opportunities.[25] Clinician fear of distraction due to interference or violence and/or obstruction of procedures were raised in four studies.[13,16,18,25]

The potential advantages and disadvantages of parent presence during invasive procedures and cardiopulmonary resuscitations according to clinicians are summarised in Table 1.

DEVELOPING EVIDENCE AND GUIDELINES

A universal call for paediatric institutions to draft guidelines and conduct clinical education has yet to occur. Hospitals that have implemented policies and initiated training programmes are more likely to permit parents to remain at the bedside.[16,18,21,23,24] Previous experience with parent presence has been reported to be associated with a more favourable clinician attitude towards the practice.[16,18,22,24] In the most recent study by Gold et al.,[20] the decision to allow family presence involved a hospital or departmental policy only 9% of the time. Even so, the study did show that 93% of clinicians would allow a parent to be present if they so wished, but the authors did not detail which situations these clinicians were referencing. It appears that clinicians' opinions towards parent presence may be shifting towards being more favourable, and more organisations are recommending that clinicians offer parents the option to stay. However, very few hospitals or departments have instituted practice guidelines or policies to assist safe and effective clinical practice during parent presence. Over 79% of clinicians have reported that they would support parent presence during complex invasive procedures and resuscitations, and more would if their institution developed a policy for this practice,[14,25] if: (i) they retained the authority to request the parents' absence at any time;[16,25] (ii) there was adequate staff to accompany the parent;[15,16,25] and (iii) there was training for clinicians to help parents cope during these events.[25] Indeed, institutional policy statements, consensus building strategies, dedicated staff resources, and education are all

Table 1 Potential advantages and disadvantages of parent presence during invasive procedures and cardiopulmonary resuscitations according to clinicians

ADVANTAGES	DISADVANTAGES
Helps calm 'sooth' the child	Risk of patient being adversely affected by parent anxiety/distress
Parents can help restrain child	Fear parent could be as complicit in painful procedures
Facilitates parent education and forges rapport	Increases the chance of performance anxiety
Enables parent to let their child know they are loved	Risk of distraction from interference/violence
Reduces suspicions, thus risk of litigation	Develops parent mistrust of healthcare provider and/or system – medicolegal concerns
Facilitates grief process	Increases risk of parent psychological traumatisation (and resulting stressful or disturbing memories)
Reduces parental procedure-related anxiety	Make teaching of junior staff more difficult
Decreases parental feelings of helplessness (increases sense of control)	Inhibits treatment by junior staff
Parents can be value added and assist with child's special needs	Requires extra time of clinician to explain procedure
Helps parent gain realistic view of care provided	Requires extra staff
Adds to parent knowledge that everything was done (peace of mind)	Constrains ability of resuscitation team to call for help

needed to move clinical practice forward in the area of parent presence.

To date, there is no evidence that directly examines the effects of supportive interventions that might facilitate parent presence. In six studies, clinicians commented on services that would be needed to encourage the implementation of parent presence during invasive procedures and resuscitations. Suggestions included educational efforts,[25] a department protocol for family presence and establishing consensus,[15,16,21,25] and dedicated family support staff.[15,16,20,21,25,27] In the one RCT, the study group relatives were all accompanied by an emergency department staff member. The designated role of these facilitators was to address the parents' emotional needs and to provide medical information, though the article did not specifically indicate how the facilitators interacted and/or helped the relatives. Family member presence carried out in this way succeeded in convincing the clinicians in this emergency department of the benefits of this practice to bereaved relatives; for that reason the pilot study was prematurely ended. Mangurten and colleagues[21] used the Emergency Nurse Association's guidelines to establish a 'family facilitator role' when providing a parent the option to be present during invasive procedures and resuscitation events. Of 36 invasive procedures and 28 resuscitations conducted with a facilitator, no patient care was recorded as being interrupted by parent presence and, overall, parents and clinicians had positive experiences with and attitudes about family presence at the beside. In the UK, where the bedside presence of parents has occurred for longer than in the US, a 1998 paediatric intensive care unit study found 46% of comments focused on the clinicians' feelings that parents were best served when accompanied by support staff to provide explanation.[16] In 2004, 93% of the UK's emergency departments that permitted family members to be present for paediatric resuscitation stated that they attempted to provide a chaperone for family members. Moreover, the lack of such a support person was cited as a reason for not permitting family presence.[15]

CHANGING MISCONCEPTIONS

If parents are not interfering with the care of their children, as several studies conclude,[14,23] then why are so many clinicians opposed to the practice? A review of the literature reveals that most parents observe quietly from a distance and/or emotionally support their child through verbal assurance or with physical contact.[21,23,26] Findings from surveys and observations have demonstrated that parents typically do not interfere with the medical care rendered to their children; in fact, their presence may actually improve the care provided. An important contribution that parents can make when present is to provide instant and important healthcare information to the clinicians during these procedures.[21]

Those ambivalent about, or opposed to, parent presence hold the position that parents may become nervous or upset during these events, which consequently may make the child and/or clinician more anxious.[13] These clinicians may worry that parents may inadvertently degrade the clinical caregiving environment by redirecting attention of the clinicians away from the child by physically or verbally interfering.[25] Parents may not comprehend what is happening to their child during these situations and, in some cases, may ask too many questions or demand attention.[13] Lastly, some researchers believe that parent presence may trigger new medicolegal issues if the outcome of the child is unfavourable or if the parents misinterpret treatment activities.[17,21,25] The literature, on the other hand, has found no studies to support these concerns.

FUTURE RESEARCH

A review of the literature not only gives an illustration of the various perspectives of parents/guardians, clinicians, and paediatric patients themselves that have been reported to date, but also encourages more research into this practice so that it can be performed safely to the benefit of parents, their children, and clinicians. More evidence is needed to describe and support the practice, particularly in the paediatric intensive care setting. Future research into the practice will determine the best methods of educating and debriefing clinicians so that the practice of parent presence can benefit both the clinicians and the parents. In addition, further study into the use, role, and cost of additional staff to support the parents would provide clinicians with a better understanding of how we can best assist parents who remain present. A more thorough investigation into the perspective of children undergoing complex invasive procedures and resuscitations would help both parents and clinicians gain more insight and skill when providing emotional and psychological support. Lastly, research is needed on the long-term effects of witnessing invasive procedures and resuscitation. Research to date has proven many acute benefits of parent presence during invasive procedure and cardiopulmonary resuscitation; however, the potential for psychological damage to parents exists, and long-term research studies must be conducted to ensure more good than harm is achieved by the practice

THE PROCESS OF PARENT-FACILITATED PRESENCE

Despite the lack of formal research regarding use of parent facilitators, experts in the field of parent presence believe it is important that institutions establish facilitator training tools and accomplish facilitator integration into the increasingly common practice of parent presence at the beside during invasive procedures and resuscitation. Such a support person may decrease variation in practice, and help staff feel better prepared to provide parents more options during these stressful events. Facilitators are to become involved after consensus has been reached by the team as to whether or not the parent(s) can be present. For clinicians who are wary of allowing parents, the nurses may suggest the use of a facilitator to care for the parent or keep them from being a disruption. A facilitator's responsibilities are multidisciplinary as they have to educate parents on the pending procedure, enable parents to be sources of comfort to their child, and care for the parents' psychosocial needs – all performed under the realm of safety for the medical team and patient. Training parent facilitators decreases variation in practice and helps staff feel better prepared to provide parents more options during these stressful events.

Key features for the implementation of parent presence practices are summarised in Boxes 1 and 2. These points are aimed at enhancing the abilities of clinicians and institutions to provide optimal care while allowing parents to remain an integral part of family-centred care during complex invasive procedures and times of emergency care.

BOX 1 Integrating the practices of parent presence during invasive procedures and cardiopulmonary resuscitation

1. Ensure commitment of the institution/department leadership to promote the practice and all protocols pertaining to it
2. Assess staff perceptions and existing practices of parent presence
3. Develop parent presence policies/guidelines
4. Provide multidisciplinary education that explains the policies/guidelines
5. Train parent facilitators and implement a code of practice during all invasive procedures and cardiopulmonary resuscitation
6. Evaluate the efficacy of the intervention and value of the practice change on the staff and patient/parent population.

Box 2 Steps to inclusion of parents during invasive procedures and cardiopulmonary resuscitation

1. Assess parental wishes, needs, and abilities and needs to be present
2. Establish team consensus regarding having the parent present
3. Designate someone to provide the parent with the option of staying or not staying in a 'non-judgmental' tone
4. Involve a parent facilitator (trained nurse, social worker, chaplain, child life therapist, physician). Facilitator is to:
   a. Provide trustworthy information to the parent as necessary and viable within the facilitators clinical realm
   b. Deal with parent's questions
   c. Provide emotional support to parents
   d. Maintain therapeutic good practice and safety
   e. Constantly assess parent's feelings, asking: 'Do you want to stay?'
   f. Advocate for the parent
   g. Know how to access resources to support families further
   h. Complete a report, documenting if parent/guardian was present and information about your role as parent facilitator
5. Continually assess clinicians' comfort with having parents present (re-establish team consensus if needed, *i.e.* new clinicians become involved in case, condition of patient changes, parents emotional state changes)
6. After each case, meet with the bedside clinicians to discuss outcomes and the effect of parent's/guardian's presence on team performance.

Key points for clinical practice

- Family-centred care embraces the idea that a parent or guardian not only meets the physical needs of their child, but also their psychosocial and developmental needs which includes being present during times of stress.

- When given the option, more parents are choosing to stay with their child during complex invasive procedures and/or resuscitations.

- Most parents do not regret experiencing their child's invasive procedure and/or resuscitation.

- There are several advantages to having parents present including: calming an anxious child, assisting in restraining a child, forging rapport between clinicians and parents, facilitating grief, reducing parental anxiety, providing urgent medical information, and confirming to the parents' that everything possible was done for their child.

- Hospitals that have implemented guidelines and/or policies and initiated training programmes in this practice are more likely to permit parents to remain safely at the bedside. *(continued)*

Key points for clinical practice *(continued)*

- Parents do not generally interfere with their child's care during invasive procedures and/or CPR. Instead, most parents are reported to either observe quietly from a distance and/or support their child emotionally through verbal re-assurance or with physical contact.

- There is little data on the paediatric patient's perspective, but some evidence suggests that parent presence was comforting to the child and is beneficial in providing help and reminding providers of their humanity.

- Parents overwhelming agree that their presence during invasive procedures and resuscitations benefits their child.

- Clinician support for parent presence remains the rate-limiting factor permitting parents to be present during complex invasive procedures and CPR, because opinions vary widely by discipline, geographic region, and hospital department.

- A designated facilitator who addresses the parents' emotional needs and provides medical information during these procedures and/or resuscitations has shown to be beneficial to the practice of parent presence.

References

1. Doyle CJ, Post H, Burney RE, Maino J, Keefe M, Rhee KJ. Family participation during resuscitation: an option. *Ann Emerg Med* 1987; **16**: 673–675.

2. Emergency Nurses Association. *Presenting the option for family presence*, 2nd edn. Park Ridge, IL: ENA, 2001.

3. American Association of Critical-Care Nurses. Practice alert: family presence during CPR and invasive procedures. *AACN News* 2004; **21**: 4.

4. American Heart Association. 2005 American Heart Association (AHA) guidelines for cardiopulmonary resuscitation (CPR) and emergency cardiovascular care (ECC) of pediatric and neonatal patients: neonatal resuscitation guidelines. *Pediatrics* 2006; **117**: e1029–e1038.

5. American Academy of Pediatrics. *PALS provider manual*. Dallas, TX: AAP 2002; 401–402.

6. Maclean SL, Guzzetta CE, White C *et al*. Family presence during cardiopulmonary resuscitation and invasive procedures: practices of critical care and emergency nurses. *J Emerg Nurs* 2003; **29**: 208–221.

7. Moyer M. Pediatric advanced life support guidelines updated, Parts 1 & 2. *Air Med J* 2002; **21**: 17–19, 26–27.

8. O'Malley P, Brown K, Mace SE. Patient- and family-centered care and the role of the emergency physician providing care to a child in the emergency department. *Pediatrics* 2006; **118**: 2242–2244.

9. Boie ET, Moore GP, Brummett C, Nelson DR. Do parents want to be present during invasive procedures performed on their children in the emergency department? A survey of 400 parents. *Ann Emerg Med* 1999; **34**: 70–74.

10. Meyers TA, Eichhorn DJ, Guzzetta CE. Do families want to be present during CPR? A retrospective survey. *J Emerg Nurs* 1998; **24**: 400–405.

11. Meyers TA, Eichhorn DJ, Guzzetta CE *et al*. Family presence during invasive procedures and resuscitation. *Am J Nurs* 2000; **100**: 32–42, quiz 43.

12. Henderson DP, Knapp JF. Report of the National Consensus Conference on Family

Presence During Pediatric Cardiopulmonary Resuscitation and Procedures. *Pediatr Emerg Care* 2005; 21: 787–791.

13. Bauchner H, Waring C, Vinci R. Parental presence during procedures in an emergency room: results from 50 observations. *Pediatrics* 1991; **87**: 544–548.

14. Powers KS, Rubenstein JS. Family presence during invasive procedures in the pediatric intensive care unit: a prospective study. *Arch Pediatr Adolesc Med* 1999; **153**: 955–958.

15. Booth MG, Woolrich L, Kinsella J. Family witnessed resuscitation in UK emergency departments: a survey of practice. *Eur J Anaesthesiol* 2004; **21**: 725–728.

16. Jarvis AS. Parental presence during resuscitation: attitudes of staff on a paediatric intensive care unit. *Intensive Crit Care Nurs* 1998; **14**: 3–7.

17. McClenathan BM, Torrington KG, Uyehara CF. Family member presence during cardiopulmonary resuscitation: a survey of US and international critical care professionals. *Chest* 2002; **122**: 2204–2211.

18. Waseem M, Ryan M. Parental presence during invasive procedures in children: what is the physician's perspective? *South Med J* 2003; **96**: 884–887.

19. Bauchner H, Vinci R, Bak S, Pearson C, Corwin MJ. Parents and procedures: a randomized controlled trial. *Pediatrics* 1996; **98**: 861–867.

20. Gold KJ, Gorenflo DW, Schwenk TL, Bratton SL. Physician experience with family presence during cardiopulmonary resuscitation in children. *Pediatr Crit Care Med* 2006; **7**: 428–433.

21. Mangurten JA, Scott SH, Guzzetta CE *et al*. Family presence: making room. *Am J Nurs* 2005; **105**: 40–48, quiz 49.

22. Sacchetti A, Carraccio C, Leva E, Harris RH, Lichenstein R. Acceptance of family member presence during pediatric resuscitations in the emergency department: effects of personal experience. *Pediatr Emerg Care* 2000; **16**: 85–87.

23. Sacchetti A, Lichenstein R, Carraccio CA, Harris RH. Family member presence during pediatric emergency department procedures. *Pediatr Emerg Care* 1996; **12**: 268–271.

24. O'Brien MM, Creamer KM, Hill EE, Welham J. Tolerance of family presence during pediatric cardiopulmonary resuscitation: a snapshot of military and civilian pediatricians, nurses, and residents. *Pediatr Emerg Care* 2002; **18**: 409–413.

25. Fein JA, Ganesh J, Alpern ER. Medical staff attitudes toward family presence during pediatric procedures. *Pediatr Emerg Care* 2004; **20**: 224–227.

26. Sacchetti A, Paston C, Carraccio C. Family members do not disrupt care when present during invasive procedures. *Acad Emerg Med* 2005; **12**: 477–479.

27. Robinson SM, Mackenzie-Ross S, Campbell Hewson GL, Egleston CV, Prevost AT. Psychological effect of witnessed resuscitation on bereaved relatives. *Lancet* 1998; **352**: 614–617.

28. Eichhorn DJ, Meyers TA, Guzzetta CE *et al*. During invasive procedures and resuscitation: hearing the voice of the patient. *Am J Nurs* 2001; **101**: 48–55.

Andre Sourander Anat Brunstein Klomek
John A Rönning

11

School bullying – a challenge and opportunity for public health interventions

DEFINITION, PREVALENCE AND INFORMANT AGREEMENT

DEVELOPMENT OF DEFINITION

The first interest in school bullying was induced in Sweden in the late 1960s by the school physician Heinemann. Although his initial focus was racial discrimination,[1] he also applied it as a general characteristic of group violence.[2] Heinemann applied the term mobbing which he had borrowed from the Austrian ethologist Konrad Lorenz.[3] From the ethologist's perspective, mobbing denoted a collective attack by a group of animals on an animal from another species, usually a natural enemy of the group. However, Lorenz also applied mobbing to characterise the action of a school class when they ganged up against a deviating individual.[3,4] Thus, at an early stage, mobbing and later bullying, was defined as a group's action towards an individual.

In the beginning of the 1970s, a change in the definition occurred with the psychologist Olweus's research on aggression. Olweus[5] was concerned that, in the original definition, the importance of the individual was overlooked. Even when mobbing was collectively induced, somebody had to initiate this collective action. Olweus was concerned that, by using the original definition, teachers would have difficulties of placing responsibility to an instigator. From Olweus's point of view, the group definition would complicate actions towards combating the phenomenon. In his later research Olweus confirmed

Andre Sourander MD (for correspondence)
Professor, Department of Child Psychiatry, Turku University Hospital, 20520 Turku, Finland
E-mail: andsou@utu.fi

Anat Brunstein Klomek PhD
Assistant Professor, Division of Child and Adolescent Psychiatry, Department of Psychiatry, Columbia University, New York, USA

John A. Rönning PhD
Department of Pediatrics, Tromsö University, Tromsö, Norway

that his early concerns had been justified.[6–8] Data from these later studies revealed that usually a relatively small number of students (two or three) in a class are involved in 50% of the incidents, and some 25% where only one is involved. These findings have been confirmed across cultures.[9] It has also been documented that a considerable percentage of students hold relatively negative attitudes about bullying see, for example, Rigby and Slee[10]).

Thus, the concept of mobbing was replaced with the concept of bullying or peer victimisation in the 1970s. The most widely employed definition is the one provided by Olweus: a person is bullied when he or she is exposed, repeatedly and over time, to negative actions on the part of one or more persons. Bullying is an intentional, aggressive act that occurs repeatedly. Olweus further suggested that bullying involves an imbalance of power. Power imbalance is used to exclude violence that is not deemed bullying. For example, if a third-grade girl is called nicknames when walking to school everyday by a younger impaired first-grader, it is not considered bullying under Olweus's definition, even though it is done deliberately and is repeated. Needless to say, there exists disagreement about including power-imbalance in the definition. Many repeated acts of violence might not be considered bullying under Olweus's definition, but would if only a behavioural definition had been used.[11,12]

Thus, there is no clear-cut understanding of how bullying should be defined. It varies with age, where younger children, 8 years and younger, tend to be more inclusive than older children, thus reporting higher rates than older children.[13] Likewise, Boulton[14] found that less than 50% of teachers and only one in five pupils in English schools defined psychological and emotional abuse as bullying. Certainly, sharing the same, or at least similar, definitions of bullying is central for accurate statistics on the incidence of bullying and for the sake of combating it.[15] There may thus be a need for operationalising what kind of acts should be included in the concept of bullying. More research and scientific debate on this issue is, therefore, warranted.

PREVALENCE AND CATEGORIES OF BULLYING

Bullying behaviour falls into four general categories: (i) direct/physical (*e.g.* assaults or theft); (ii) direct/verbal (*e.g.* threats, insults or nicknames); (iii) indirect/relational (*e.g.* social exclusion, spreading nasty rumours); and (iv) the newest form, cyber.

Cyberbullying manifests itself through annoying and intimidating messages. They may come in the form of private text messages or e-mails, pictures posted without permission (especially embarrassing photographs), and rumours spread via e-mail, text messages, telephone calls and social networking Web sites like Facebook.com and MySpace.com.[16]

The latest, large-scale, international comparison was carried out on national representative samples in 28 countries in Europe and North America, involving 123,227 students aged 11, 13, and 15 years of age.[17] The proportion of students being bullied varied enormously across countries. The lowest prevalence was reported among girls in Sweden (6.3%), the highest among boys in Lithuania (41.4%). Generally, girls were less involved in bullying behaviours than boys. Most studies report on school-aged children, especially youths. Very few studies have been carried out on younger children. However, conducting interviews with 1982 children aged 6–9 years Wolke and colleagues[18] labelled 4.3% as direct bullies, 39,8% as victims, and 10.2% as both bullies and victims. The rates for relational bullying were 1.1% bullies, 37.9% victims and 5.9% bully/victims. Boys were rated more often as both direct and relational bullies, victims and bully/victims than girls. In a study involving 344 5–7-year-olds in kindergarten, Perren and Alsaker[19] were able to identify victims, bullies and bully-victims. In future studies on 'traditional' bullying, there is a need to differentiate distinctly between categories of bullying and to specify gender. This is of great importance in order to evaluate whether some types of bullying have differential adverse effects on gender. For the sake of prevention and early intervention, more research should study pre-school samples.

Research on cyberbullying is at a very early stage. However, a recent study[16] found cyberbullying to be less frequent than traditional bullying, and reported more outside of school than inside. Telephone call and text message bullying were most prevalent, students perceiving their impact as comparable to traditional bullying. Although rarer, mobile phone/video clip bullying was perceived to have the most negative impact.

CROSS-INFORMANT AGREEMENT OF BULLYING

Clinicians and researchers accept that it is necessary to collect data from multiple sources, such as parents, teachers, and children themselves, to obtain a comprehensive and accurate picture of children's adjustment.[20] High agreement between informants about bullying would thus mean high validity about which children should be targeted for intervention and prevention procedures. Numerous studies have examined cross-informant correlations regarding psychopathology, and uncovered low agreement.[20–22] The Finnish nation-wide 'From a Boy to a Man' study, a follow-up study included in the Epidemiological Multicentre Child Psychiatric Study in Finland, is the only longitudinal population-based study examining agreement between bullying and victimisation among children, parents and teachers. Information from 2713 boys about bullying and victimisation at the age of 8 years was correlated with information about psychiatric disorders at 18–23 years of age. Agreement between informants was poor. Teachers reported higher levels of frequent bullying than others, whereas children reported the highest percentage of victimisation. However, all three informant groups' reports of 'frequent bullying' predicted later psychiatric disorder. Teachers' reports of 'frequent victimisation' were the strongest predictors of later psychiatric disorder. From the point of view of early problem recognition this is important, and offers further support to earlier arguments that the education system, and school healthcare in mid-childhood, are of central importance in the early detection of later social maladjustment.[23,24] Informants' reports about 'infrequent bullying' showed, at most, a rather low risk of adverse outcome.

As expected, teachers reported a particularly high level of 'frequent bullying' (7%) compared to the children themselves (2%) and parents (1%). The finding that teachers report such a high percentage of frequent bullying compared to the children themselves is interesting, in light of the fact that incidents of aggression and bullying in the school are often subtle, indirect, and not easily observable by teachers.[25] On the other hand, the difference in proportion between teacher and child concerning bullying could mean that children's lower report is a reflection of bullying being a socially undesirable act. Children identified as aggressors may be less likely than others to identify aggressive acts as bullying.[26] Thus, these individuals may downplay or justify their bullying behaviour by not identifying it as bullying.[27]

BULLYING AND HEALTH PROBLEMS

BULLYING AND PSYCHIATRIC PROBLEMS

Bullying and victimisation are associated with poorer family functioning,[28] interparental violence,[29] and parental maltreatment.[30] Bullies have been found to be aggressive, hostile, and domineering toward peers; to score higher on conduct and hyperactivity symptoms; and to show little anxiety or insecurity. Victims tend to be more depressed, withdrawn, anxious, and insecure; to score higher on internalising and psychosomatic scales; to show lower levels of self-esteem; and to be more cautious, sensitive, and quieter than other students.[31–33]

Previous studies have suggested that bully-victims are the most troubled in terms of outcomes.[34–36] Like bullies, they display high levels of physical and verbal aggression. They score high on measures of both externalising and hyperactive behaviour but low on measures of self-worth, academic competence, and social acceptance.[32,37,38] In contrast to the more goal-oriented aggression of bullies, bully-victims' aggression is considered to be a reflection of an underlying state of poorly modulated anger and irritability.

Based on cross-sectional studies, bullying and peer victimisation appear to be linked to depression.[39–41] In studies examining the relationship between bullying and depression, victims are found to manifest more depressive symptoms and psychological distress compared to non-victims.[32,34,41–43] Findings pertaining to bullies are less consistent. Some studies did not find an association between being a bully and depression whereas others have found that bullies, and not just victims, report high levels of depression.[34,39,40,44] These inconsistent results may be explained by a different threshold in which bullying is associated with depression and suicide risk among females and males.[40] Those who are both victims and bullies are usually found to be at the highest risk for depression.[39,40]

To date, most of our empirical knowledge of the effects of bullying is based on cross-sectional studies. Usually, only symptom questionnaires were used, frequently using only one informant. Only a few population-based studies have examined the effects of bullying prospectively. Bond et al.[45] showed that victimisation at age 13 years predicted the onset of self-reported symptoms of anxiety and depression 1 year later. Arsenault et al.[46] found that victims and bully-victims showed more behavioural and school adjustment problems at 7 years of age, even after controlling for pre-existing adjustment problems at the age of 5 years, in a nationally representative cohort study. In a Korean study, Kim et al.[35] followed seventh- and eighth-grade students for 10 months and showed that problem behaviour was a consequence, rather than a cause, of bullying experience. Kumpulainen et al.[34] found that bullying at 8 years of age was associated with later psychiatric symptoms in pre-adolescence. Bullying and being bullied are found to be rather stable between the ages of 8 and 16 years. In a Finnish cohort, almost all boys who were bullied at the age of 16 years had been bullied already at age 8 years. Half of the boys who bullied at 16 years had already been bullying as 8-year-olds. Furthermore, bullying at age 8 years strongly predicted criminality in adolescence.[36]

In the Finnish 'From a boy to a man' study, information about bullying and victimisation was gathered in 1989 when the boys were 8 years old from parents, teachers, and children. Information about psychiatric disorders was based on military call-up examination and army registry when the subjects were 18–23 years old.[23] The findings suggest that both bullying and victimisation during early school years are public health signs that can identify boys who are at risk of suffering psychiatric disorders in early adulthood. When controlled for the effect of parental education level and general emotional and behavioural symptomatology, frequent victimisation independently predicted anxiety disorders and frequent bullying predicted antisocial personality disorder, whereas frequent bully-victimisation predicted both of these disorders. However, bullies and victims with psychiatric symptoms at age 8 years rather than all bullies or victims *per se* were are at elevated risk of later psychiatric disorders. If the frequent bully or victim did not have a high level of symptoms at age 8 years, results from the 'From a boy to a man' study suggest that the primary intervention focus should be on regulating the child's behaviour at school and enhancing peer relationships. An approach of screening that relies first on identifying frequent bullies, victims, or bully-victims, and then conducts a psychiatric screening could be a cost-effective alternative to universal screening of all children for psychiatric problems, especially when child mental health resources are scarce. However, the screening approach requires second-stage clinical evaluations, effectively functioning child mental health services, and efforts to assist families in obtaining help.

BULLYING AND SUICIDE

Based on cross-sectional studies, bullying and peer victimisation also appear to be linked to the idea of suicide[39–41,44,48,49] and suicide attempts.[39,40,48] A recent publication by Kim and Leventhal[50] has systematically reviewed studies conducted in children and adolescents that examined the association between bullying and suicide. The review indicated that any participation in bullying increases the risk of thoughts of suicide and/or suicidal behaviour. There are significant interactions between gender and bullying in the risk of suicide.[40,41,44,48]

In a recent Finnish longitudinal study,[51] we found that childhood bullying behaviour among 8-year-old boys is a risk factor for later depression but the association between bullying others and thoughts of suicide became non-significant after controlling for depression at age 8 years. A current longitudinal study aims to examine the association between childhood bullying with later suicide attempts and completed suicide among both genders.[52]

BULLYING AND CRIMINALITY

Bullying is a component of an antisocial, rule-breaking pattern of behaviour.[53] In a cross-sectional US study, Nansel et al.[54] found a strong and consistent relationship between bullying and involvement in violent behaviour. Bullies engage in high rates of interpersonal power dominance and instrumental aggression such as coercing others to give them their property. Longitudinal studies show that this type of behaviour pattern (i.e. externalising problems) is relatively stable over time. Aggressive trajectories are associated with subsequent antisocial and criminal behaviour in adolescence.[55,56] Age at onset as well as level and form of aggression have become important factors in understanding antisocial development, as early onset of antisocial behaviour is regarded as a reliable predictor of adult antisocial behaviour.

The results from the Finnish 'From a boy to a man' cohort study show that frequent bullying in childhood predicts criminality in late adolescence. Boys who bully frequently in childhood are at elevated risk for recidivism and for committing violent, property, traffic, and drunk-driving offences in late adolescence.[36] To illustrate this, 21.1% of frequent bully-victims and 15.9% of those with frequent bully-only status were recidivist offenders, compared with only 6.8% of those who did not exhibit frequent bullying behaviour. Although frequent bullies and bully-victims composed only 8.8% of the total sample, they were responsible for 33.0% of all offences during the 4-year period between the ages of 16 and 20 years (i.e. 8–12 years after the initial assessment). These results have considerable significance for the early prevention of criminality, indicating that early crime prevention that focuses on bullying should be one of the highest priorities in child public health policy. Frequent bullying may serve as an important red flag that something is wrong and that intensive preventive or ameliorative interventions are warranted. In contrast, being a frequent victim does not appear to be related to significant later delinquency and aggression but may instead involve internalising and covert behaviour (including property offences) rather than crimes directed against other people.

BULLYING AND PSYCHOSOMATIC PROBLEMS

Fewer studies have been conducted regarding the relationship of bullying behaviour and physical health, compared to studies on the relationship between involvement in bullying and mental health. One of the first studies of this relationship examined 2962 primary school children in London,[58] and found significantly more self-reported physical problems among bullied students. Victimised children were more likely to have sleeping problems, bed wetting, headaches, and stomach aches. An Australian study[59] of high-school students revealed that boys and girls experiencing high levels of victimisation early in high school had significantly poorer physical health later, even after controlling for physical health during the first assessment. Finally, a Dutch study[60] following 1118 children aged 9–11 years on two occasions found that victims of bullying had significantly higher chances of developing new psychosomatic and psychosocial problems compared to children who were not bullied. However, some psychosocial, but not physical health, symptoms preceded bullying victimisation. Although the follow-up periods in the two last studies were relatively short, both indicated that bullying and victimisation cause physical health problems. Surely, longer prospective studies are warranted starting in the preschool years. Nevertheless, findings such as these stress the importance for physicians and health practitioners to screen whether bullying plays a role in the aetiology of physical symptoms.

BULLYING AND OBESITY

The prevalence of childhood obesity is rapidly increasing and has doubled in the last two decades, making it one of the most challenging public health issues of our time.[61,62] Childhood obesity is associated with many clinical health problems such as type 2 diabetes and cardiovascular disease;[63,64] in addition, obese children are more likely to become obese adults having an increased risk of morbidity and mortality in adulthood.[65] Childhood obesity is also associated with many negative psychological and social consequences such as impaired peer relationships, school experiences, and poor psychological well-being. However, few studies have investigated the relationship between obesity and bullying. The study of Griffiths et al.[66] included a 1-year follow-up from age 7.5 to 8.5 years and concluded that obesity is predictive of bullying involvement for both boys and girls. Young adolescents are more likely to be targets of bullying because they deviate from appearance ideals. However, obese boys are more likely to be bullies, presumably because of their physical dominance in the peer group. For health practitioners treating obese children, it would thus be of the upmost importance to assess bullying and victimisation in their lives in order to promote effective life-style changes.

INTERVENTION STUDIES

General

A growing number of world-wide studies have examined interventions targeted to reduce bullying behaviours.[67,68] Research on the effectiveness of school bullying interventions has lagged behind descriptive studies on this topic. Although the literature on bullying intervention research has only recently expanded to a point that allows for meta-analysis, research has not reached a point to allow identification of the essential elements of the programmes nor how interventions should be implemented. The intervention programmes vary in their effectiveness of reducing bullying behaviour at school.

The first widely disseminated published research on school bullying interventions was the work of Olweus.[53,70,71] The Olweus Bullying Prevention Program is a multilevel, multicomponent school-based programme designed to prevent or reduce bullying in elementary, middle, and junior high schools (ages 6–15 years). Olweus's intervention has been the blue-print for other interventions around the world. The Olweus programme works with interventions at three levels – school, classroom, and individuals involved. Evaluation of the Olweus Bullying Prevention Program report reductions of 30–70% in the student reports of being bullied and bullying others.[53,70,71] However, evaluation of similar prevention programmes implemented in other countries seem less promising (see, for example, Roland[72] and Stevens et al.[73]).

There have been a limited number of reviews published in the last few years focusing on bullying interventions. The review by Smith et al.[74] focused on whole-school antibullying programmes and was based on 14 studies. The authors concluded that only some interventions had positive outcomes while most of programmes had non-significant outcomes on self-report measures of bullying and victimisation. They also found that programmes in which implementation was systematically monitored tended to be more effective than those without any monitoring. One limitation of this study is that many bullying interventions are not whole-school intervention but are implemented with small groups of students.

Menell et al.[69] conducted a meta-analysis of school bullying intervention research from 1980 to 2004. The review included 16 intervention studies with 15,386 student participants from Europe and the US. Contrary to the study by Smith et al.,[74] Mennel et al.[69] evaluated both studies that focused on whole-school interventions and studies targeting smaller groups in the schools. They concluded that the interventions did not dramatically reduce the incidence of bullying and victimisation behaviour. However, the interventions were more likely to influence knowledge, attitudes, and self-perceptions. Specifically, the interventions enhanced students' social competence, self-esteem, and peer acceptance and also enhanced teachers' knowledge of effective practices, feelings of efficacy regarding intervention skills, and actual behaviour in responding to incidences of bullying at school. Their findings indicated that the majority of intervention effects did not demonstrate sufficient power to be considered meaningful or clinically important. Although few interventions were associated with negative effects, the authors believe that school bullying interventions do not harm students. The negative findings may be sample specific or could be attributed to something other than the intervention.

Mennel et al.[69] found a stronger pattern of meaningful positive effects across studies compared to Smith and colleagues.[74] The different findings may be attributed to the broader literature base of the Mennel et al.[69] study and the fact that it was not limited to whole-school programmes. A limitation of the review by Mennell et al.[69] is that the studies included varied widely in terms of research design, intervention models, and intensity of intervention.

Vreeman and Carroll[76] also conducted a systematic review of rigorously evaluated school-based interventions to decrease bullying. The review included 26 interventions for primary school students, and the students' grade-levels varied from first to eighth grade. The types of intervention were categorised into five groups: curriculum interventions, multidisciplinary or whole-school interventions, targeted social and behavioural skills groups, mentoring, and increased social work support. Based on their categorisation, we describe the three main categories of interventions – whole-school interventions, curriculum interventions, and social and behavioural skills groups.

Whole-school interventions

In whole-school interventions, bullying is considered a systemic problem that requires a systemic approach implemented throughout the school. These programmes attempt to restructure the whole school environment to reduce opportunities and rewards for bullying. The interventions target different levels of the school organisation, and include multiple disciplines. The interventions usually involve individuals, classrooms, teachers, and administration staff. They also include clear and consistent policies, rules and sanctions against bullying (*e.g.* zero tolerance for bullying behaviour), staff and parent training, classroom interventions and individual level interventions. Most researchers agree that most effective programmes are comprehensive.

The most widely evaluated bullying intervention programme in the world is the Olweus Bullying Prevention Program.[53,70,71] This pioneered the whole-school approach to preventing and reducing bullying with an intervention programme in Norway. The intervention includes training for school personnel, materials for parents, a video-taped classroom curriculum, and evaluation using the Olweus Bully/Victim Questionnaire (filled out anonymously by the students).[77] The evaluation indicated decreased bullying, victimisation, and antisocial behaviour, as well as improved school climate.[71,77] The Olweus intervention has been implemented in several other countries. Overall, these whole-school studies had positive effects on bullying. Of eight studies, seven revealed positive outcomes.[78–84] Five of these studies reported decreases in bullying or victimisation.[78–80,82,84] The evaluation of the Olweus Bullying Prevention Program in Rogaland, Norway, however,[72] has resulted in less promising results.

Whole-school interventions more often reduce victimisation and bullying than interventions that only include classroom-level curricula or social skills groups.[76] The success of the whole-school interventions indicates that bullying involves social factors which are external to individual children's psychosocial problems. Despite the evidence pointing toward the value of whole-school approaches, significant barriers may still limit their effectiveness; for example, the specific school environment could significantly impact effectiveness. In addition, sometimes the specific components of an intervention are not always described sufficiently to enable good replication.

Curriculum interventions

Curriculum interventions aim to promote an antibullying attitude within the classroom and to help children develop prosocial conflict resolution skills. Most of these interventions focus on changing students' attitudes and group norms as well as increasing self-efficacy. The curriculum interventions include video-tapes, lectures, and written curriculum, and vary in intensity. Curriculum changes are often attractive because they usually require smaller resources, personnel, and effort.

In the review by Vreeman and Carroll,[76] curriculum interventions did not consistently decrease bullying, and several actually suggested that the bullying within the intervention group increased. Of the 10 studies of curriculum interventions, six showed no significant improvements in bullying.[73,85–87] Of the four studies that did show less bullying after a curriculum intervention, three also showed more bullying or victimisation in certain populations or with certain measurement tools.[85,88,89] The study by Baldry and Farrington[85] showed a decrease in self-reported victimisation among older children, but younger children actually reported more victimisation, and there were no significant differences in either victimisation or bullying overall.

Social and behavioural skills group interventions

The social and behavioural skills group training interventions are also based on social, cognitive and behavioural changes. Social skills training helps bullying or victimised children learn to change their attitudes and behaviour. Four studies[90–93] providing training in social skills did not clearly improve bullying or victimisation. The DeRosier[90] report was the only social skills training intervention that showed clear reductions in bullying from the intervention. Older children had worse outcomes from the social skills training groups than younger children.[90] The other social skills group interventions, all of which involved older children, did not result in clear changes. The failure of these interventions points again to the inability of a single-level intervention to reduce bullying significantly. Overall, these studies suggest that failing to address the whole school and social environment undermines success.

CONCLUSIONS

Bullying is an aspect of a serious antisocial trajectory that is rather stable over time. Bullying may signal an elevated risk of later psychiatric problems and committing crimes, but the child's behaviour needs to be assessed in its entirety. Particular attention should be paid to children who display frequent bullying behaviour, and especially to frequent bully-victims because they are at risk of developing later adverseries. Because childhood bullying is complex with potentially serious consequences, the early identification of children-at-risk should be a priority for society. In addition to the personal costs and pain these children bring to their fellow human beings and themselves, their serious and persistent problems result in huge public cost. Greater investment in prevention systems and procedures in children's natural environments such as the home, kindergarten, and school could be of immense benefit to society.

There is a body of evidence that school-based intervention programmes can be effective in reducing the level of school bullying. However, not all programmes have proved effective. An intervention at only one level is unlikely to have a significant impact. The chance of success is greater if the intervention incorporates a whole-school approach involving multiple disciplines. The use of curriculum or targeted social skills groups alone less often results in a decrease in bullying and sometimes even worsens bullying and victimisation. Intervention can succeed, but not enough is known to indicate exactly how and when. Additional research on antibullying interventions is clearly needed.

Key points for clinical practice

- A person is bullied when he or she is exposed, repeatedly and over time, to negative actions on the part of one or more persons.

- Bullying behaviour falls into four general categories: direct/physical, direct/verbal, indirect/relational and cyber.

- Informant agreement about bullying between students, teachers and parents is poor. Teacher report best predicts later psychiatric problems.

- Based on cross-sectional studies, bullying and peer victimisation appear to be linked to psychopathology including depression and risk of suicide.

- Bullying is also associated with health and psychosomatic problems.

- Findings from a Finnish birth cohort study show that both bullying and victimisation during early school years are public health signs that can identify boys who are at risk of suffering psychiatric disorders in early adulthood.

- Boys who bully frequently in childhood are at elevated risk for crime recidivism and for committing violent, property, traffic, and drunk-driving offences in late adolescence.

- Boys who both bully and are victimised (*i.e.* bully-victims) are the most troubled in terms of outcomes.

- According to the Finnish birth cohort study, bullies and victims with psychiatric symptoms at age 8 years rather than all bullies or victims per se are at elevated risk of later psychiatric disorders.

- An approach to screening that relies first on identifying frequent bullies, victims, or bully-victims, and then conducts a psychiatric screening could be a cost-effective alternative to universal screening of all children for psychiatric problems, especially when child mental health resources are scarce.

- Frequent bullying may serve as an important red flag that something is wrong and that intensive preventive or ameliorative interventions are warranted.

- Compared to frequent bullying, infrequent bullying showed a rather low risk of adverse outcome.

- A growing number of studies have examined interventions targeted to reduce bullying behaviour at school.

- The three main categories of interventions are: whole-school interventions, curriculum interventions, and social and behavioural skills groups.

- The intervention programmes vary in their effectiveness of reducing bullying behaviour at school.

- Comprehensive whole-school interventions are usually more effective than a single-level intervention.

- More research is needed to understand the essential elements of the programmes and how interventions should be implemented.

References

1. Heinemann P-P. Apartheid. *Liberal debatt* 1969; **2**: 3–14.
2. Heinemann P-P. *Gruppvåld bland barn och vuxna* [Group violence among children and adults]. Stockholm: Nature och Kultur, 1973.
3. Lorenz K. *On Aggression*. New York: Harcourt, Brace and World, 2001.
4. Olweus D. Peer harassment. a critical analysis and some important issues. In: Juvonen G. (ed) *Peer harassment in school. The plight of the vulnerable and victimized*. New York: Guilford Press, 1966; 3–20.
5. Olweus D. *Hackkycklingar och översittare. Forskning om skolmobbing*. Stockholm: Almquist & Wicksell, 1973.
6. Olweus D. *Aggression in schools: bullies and whipping boys*. Washington, DC: Hemisphere Press (Wiley), 1978.
7. Olweus D. Stability of aggressive reaction patterns in males: a review. *Psychol Bull* 1979; **86**: 852–875.
8. Olweus D, Solberg M. *Cross-cultural study of bully/victim problems in school: final report for Norway to Japanese Ministry of Education*. Tokyo: Japanese Ministry of Education, 1998.
9. Smith PK, Morita Y, Junger-Tas J *et al. The Nature of School Bullying. A Cross-National Perspective*. New York: Routledge, 1999.
10. Rigby K, Slee P. Bullying among Australian school children: reported behaviour and attitudes to victims. *J Soc Psychol* 1991; **131**: 615–627.
11. Aalsma MC, Brown JR. What is bullying? [Editorial] *J Adolesc Health* 2008; **43**: 101–102.
12. Sawyer AL, Bradshaw CP, O'Brennan LM. Examining ethnic, gender, and development differences in the way children report being a victim of 'bullying' on self-report measures. *J Adolesc Health* 2008; **43**: 106–114.
13. Smith PK, Cowie H, Olafsson RF, Liefooghe APD. Definitions of bullying: a comparison of terms used, and age and gender differences, in a fourteen-country international comparison. *Child Dev* 2002; **73**:1119–1133.
14. Boulton MJ. Teachers' view on bullying definitions, attitudes and ability to cope. *Br J Educ Psychol* 1997; **67**: 223–233.
15. Rønning JA, Sourander A, Kumpulainen K *et al.* Cross-informant agreement about bullying and victimization among eight-year-olds: whose information best predicts psychiatric caseness 10–15 years later? *Soc Psychiatry Psychiatric Epidemiol* 2008 (Pubmed ahead of print).
16. Smith PK, Mahdavi J, Carvalho M *et al.* Cyberbullying: its nature and impact in secondary school pupils. *J Child Psychol Psychiatry* 2008; **49**: 376–385.
17. Due P, Holstein BE, Lynch J *et al.* The Health Behaviour in School-Aged Children Bully Working Group. Bullying and symptoms among school-aged children: international comparative cross sectional study in 28 countries. *Eur J Public Health* 2005; **15**: 128–132.
18. Wolke D, Woods S, Blomfield L, Karstadt L. The association between direct and relational bullying and behaviour problems among primary school children. *J Child Psychol Psychiatry* 2000; **41**: 989–1002.
19. Perren S, Alsaker FD. Social behavior and peer relationships of victims, bully-victims, and bullies in kindergarten. *J Child Psychol Psychiatry* 2006; **47**: 45–57.
20. Achenbach TM, McConaughy SH, Howell CT. Child/adolescent behavioural and emotional problems: implications of cross-informant correlations for situational specificity. *Psychol Bull* 1987; **101**: 213–232.
21. Sourander A, Helselä L, Helenius H. Parent-adolescent agreement on emotional and behavioural problems. *Soc Psychiatry Psychiatr Epidemiol* 1999; **34**: 657–663.
22. Verhulst FC, Dekker MC, van der Ende J. Parent, teacher and self-reports as predictors of signs of disturbance in adolescents: whose information carries the most weight? *Acta Psychiatr Scand* 1997; **96**: 75–81.
23. Sourander A, Jensen P, Rønning JA *et al.* What is the early adulthood outcome of boys who bully or are bullied in childhood? The Finnish 'From a boy to a man' study. *Pediatrics* 2007; **120**: 397–404.
24. Sourander A, Jensen P, Rønning JA *et al.* Are childhood bullies and victims at risk of criminality in late adolescence? The Finnish 'From a boy to a man' study. *Arch Pediatr Adolesc Med* 2007; **161**: 546–552.

25. Owens L, Shute R, Slee P. Guess what I just heard!; indirect aggression among teenage girls in Australia. *Aggressive Behav* 2000; **26**: 67–83.

26. Monks CP, Smith PK. Definitions of bullying: age differences in understanding of the term, and the role of experience. *Br J Dev Psychol* 2006; **24**: 801–821.

27. Boulton MJ, Trueman M, Flemington I. Associations between secondary school pupils' definitions of bullying, attitudes towards bullying, and tendencies to engage in bullying: age and sex differences. *Educ Studies* 2002; **28**: 353–370.

28. Rigby K, Cox I, Black G. Cooperativeness and bully/victim problems among Australian school children. *J Soc Psychol* 1997; **137**: 357–368.

29. Baldry AC. Bullying in schools and exposure to domestic violence. *Child Abuse Neglect* 2003; **27**: 713–732.

30. Shields A, Cicchetti D. Parental maltreatment and emotion dysregulation as risk factors for bullying and victimization in middle childhood. *J Clin Child Psychol* 2001; **30**: 349–363.

31. Craig WM. The relationship among bullying, victimization, depression, anxiety and aggression in elementary school children. *Personality Individual Differences* 1998; **24**: 123–130.

32. Kumpulainen K, Räsänen E, Henttonen I *et al*. Bullying and psychiatric symptoms among elementary school-age children. *Child Abuse Neglect* 1998; **22**: 705–717.

33. Olweus D. Bullying or peer abuse at school: facts and intervention. *Curr Direct Psychol Sci* 1995; **4**: 196–200.

34. Kumpulainen K, Räsänen E. Children involved in bullying at elementary school age: their psychiatric symptoms and deviance in adolescence: an epidemiological sample. *Child Abuse Neglect* 2000; **24**: 1567–1577.

35. Kim YS, Leventhal BL, Koh YJ, Hubbard A, Boyce AT. School bullying and youth violence: causes or consequences of psychopathology? *Arch Gen Psychiatry* 2006; **63**: 1035–1041.

36. Sourander A, Jensen P, Ronning JA *et al*. Childhood bullies and victims and their risk of criminality in late adolescence. *Arch Pediatr Adolesc Med* 2007; **161**: 546–552.

37. Austin S, Joseph S. Assessment of bully/victim problems in 8- to 11-year-olds. *Br J Educ Psychol* 1996; **66**: 447–456.

38. Woods S, White E. The association between bullying behaviour, arousal levels and behaviour problems. *J Adolesc* 2005; **28**: 381–395.

39. Kaltiala-Heino R, Rimpela M, Marttunen M, Rimpela A, Rantanen P. Bullying, depression, and suicidal ideation in Finnish adolescents: school survey. *BMJ* 1999; **319**: 348–351.

40. Brunstein Klomek A, Sourander A, Kumpulainen K, *et al*. Childhood bullying as a risk for later depression and suicidal ideation among Finnish males. *J Affect Disord* 2008; **109**(1–2): 47–55.

41. van der Wal M, de Wit C, Hirasing, R. Psychosocail health among young victims and offenders of direct and indirect bullying. *Pediatrics* 2003; **111**: 1312–1317.

42. Mills C, Guerin S, Lynch F, Daly I, Fitzpatrick C. The relationship between bullying, depression and suicidal thoughts/behavior in Irish adolescents. *Irish J Psychol Med* 2004; **21**: 112–116.

43. Williams K, Chambers M, Logan S, Robinson D, Association of common health symptoms with bullying in primary school children. *BMJ* 1996; **313**: 17–19.

44. Roland E. Bullying, depressive symptoms and suicidal thoughts. *Educ Res* 2002; **44**: 55–67.

45. Bond L, Carlin JB, Thomas L, Rubin K, Patton G. Does bullying cause emotional problems? A prospective study of young teenagers. *BMJ* 2001; **323**: 480–484.

46. Arsenault L, Walsh E, Trzesniewski K *et al*. Bullying victimization uniquely contributes to adjustment problems in young children: a nationally representative cohort study. *Pediatrics* 2006; **118**: 130–138.

47. Sourander A, Helstelä L, Helenius H, Piha J. Persistence of bullying from childhood to adolescence: a longitudinal 8-year follow-up study. *Child Abuse Neglect* 2000; **24**: 873–881.

48. Kim YS, Koh YJ, Leventhal BL. School bullying and suicidal risk in Korean middle school students. *Pediatrics* 2005; **115**: 357–363.

49. Rigby K, Slee P. Suicidal ideation among adolescent school children, involvement in

bully-victim problems and perceived social support. *Suicide Life-Threatening Behav* 1999; **29**: 119–130.

50. Kim YS, Leventhal B. Bullying and suicide. A review. *Int J Adolesc Med Health* 2008; **20**: 133–154.

51. Brunstein Klomek A, Sourander A, Kumpulainen K *et al*. Childhood bullying as a risk for later depression and suicidal ideation among Finnish males. *J Affect Disord* 2008; **109**: 47–55.

52. Brunstein Klomek A, Sourander A , Niemelä S, Kumpulainen K *et al*. Childhood Bullying Behaviors as a Risk for Suicide Attempts and Completed Suicides: A Population-Based Birth Cohort Study. *J Am Acad Child Adolesc Psychiatry* 2008; In press.

53. Olweus D. *Bullying at School: What We Know and What We Can Do*. Cambridge, MA: Blackwell, 1993.

54. Nansel TR, Overpeck MD, Haynie DL, Ruan WJ, Scheidt P. Relationships between bullying and violence among US youth. *Arch Pediatr Adolesc Med* 2003; **157**: 348–353.

55. Maughan B, Pickles A, Rowe R, Costello EJ, Angold A. Developmental trajectories of aggressive and nonaggressive conduct problems. *J Quant Criminol* 2000; **16**: 199–221.

56. Nagin D, Tremblay RE. Trajectories of boys' physical aggression, opposition, and hyperactivity on the path to physically violent and nonviolent juvenile delinquency. *Child Dev* 1999; **70**: 1181–1196.

57. Moffitt TE, Caspi A, Harrington H, Milne BJ. Males on the life-course-persistent and adolescence-limited antisocial pathways: follow-up at age 26 years. *Dev Psychopathol* 2002; **14**: 179–207.

58. Williams K, Chambers M, Logan S, Robinson D. Associations of common health symptoms with bullying in primary school children. *BMJ* 1996; **313**: 17–19.

59. Rigby K. Peer victimization at school and the health of secondary school students. *Br J Educ Psychol* 1999; **69**: 95–104.

60. Fekkes M, Pijpers FIM, Fredriks AM, Vogels T, Verloove-Vanhorick SP. Do bullied children get ill, or do ill children get bullied? A prospective cohort study on the relationship between bullying and health-related symptoms. *Pediatrics* 2006; **117**: 1568–1574.

61. Bundred PD, Kitchiner D, Buchan I. Prevalence of overweight and obese children between 1989 and 1998: population based series of cross sectional studies. *BMJ* 2001; **322**: 1–4.

62. Relly JJ, Dorosty AR. Epidemic of obesity in UK children. *Lancet* 1999; **354**: 1–4.

63. Fagot-Campagna A, Saaddine JB, Flegal KM, Beckles GL. Diabetes, impaired fasting glucose, and elevated HbA1c in U.S. adolescents and the Third National Health and Nutrition Examination Survey. *Diabetes Care* 2001; **24**: 834–837.

64. Sinha R, Fisch G, Teague B *et al*. Prevalence of impaired glucose tolerance among children and adolescents with marked obesity. *N Engl J Med* 2002; **346**: 802–810.

65. Freedman DS, Khan LK, Dietz WH, Srinivasan SR, Berenson GS. Relationship of childhood obesity to coronary heart disease risk factors in adulthood: the Bogalusa Heart Study. *Pediatrics* 2001; **108**: 712–718.

66. Griffiths LJ, Wolke D, Page JP, Horwood JP, the ALSPAC Study Team. Obesity and bullying: different effects for boys and girls. *Arch Dis Child* 2006; **91**: 121–125.

67. Rigby K, Slee PT. Australia. In: Smith PK, Morita Y, Junger-tas J, Olweus D, Catalano R, Slee P. (eds) *The nature of school bullying. A cross-national perspective*. London: Routledge, 1999; 324–340.

68. Pepler D, Craig W, Ziegler S, Charach A. An evaluation of an anti-bullying intervention in Toronto schools. *Can J Community Mental Health* 1994; **13**: 95–110.

69. Menell KW, Gueldner BA, Ross SW, Isava DM. How Effective Are School Bullying Intervention Programs? A Meta-Analvsis of Intervention Research. *School Psychology* 2008; **23**(1): 26–42.

70. Olweus D. Bully/victim problems among schoolchildren: basic facts and effects of a school based intervention program. In: Pepler DJ, Rubin KH *et al*. (eds) *The development and treatment of childhood aggression*. Hillsdale: Lawrence Erlbaum, 1991; 411–448.

71. Olweus D. Bullying at school: basic facts and an effective intervention programme. *Promotion Educ* 1994; **1**: 27–31, 48.

72. Roland E. Bullying in school: three national innovations in Norwegian schools in 15 years. *Aggressive Behav* 2000; **26**: 135–143.

73. Stevens V, De Bourdeaudhuij I, Van Oost P. Bullying in Flemish schools: an evaluation of anti-bullying intervention in primary and secondary schools. *Br J Educ Psychol* 2000; **70**: 195–210.

74. Smith JD, Schneider BH, Smith PK, Ananiadou K. The effectiveness of whole school antibullying programs A: synthesis of evaluation research. *School Psychol Rev* 2004; **33**: 547–560.

75. Leadbetter B, Hoglund W, Woods T. Changing contexts? The effects of a primary prevention program on classroom levels of peer relational and physical victimization. *J Community Psychol* 2003; **31**: 397–418.

76. Vreeman RC, Carroll AE. A systematic review of school-based interventions to prevent bullying. *Arch Pediatr Adolesc Med* 2007; **161**: 78–88.

77. Olweus D. Bullying among school children: intervention and prevention. In: Peters RD, McMahon RJ, Quinsey VL. (eds) *Aggression and Violence Throughout the Life Span*. London: Sage Publications, 1992; 100–125.

78. Alsaker FD, Valkanover S. Early diagnosis and prevention of victimization in kindergarten. In: Juvonen J, Graham S. (eds) *Peer Harassment in School*. New York, NY: Guilford Press, 2001; 175–195.

79. Menesini E, Codecasa E, Benelli B, Cowie H. Enhancing children's responsibility to take action against bullying: evaluation of a befriending intervention in Italian middle schools. *Aggressive Behav* 2003; **29**: 1–14.

80. Metzler C, Biglan A, Rusby J, Sprague J. Evaluation of a comprehensive behavior management program to improve school-wide positive behavior support. *Educ Treatment Child* 2001; **24**: 448–479.

81. Mitchell J, Palmer S, Booth M, Powell Davies G. A randomised trial of an intervention to develop health promoting schools in Australia: the south western Sydney study. *Aust NZ J Public Health* 2000; **24**: 242–246.

82. Rahey L, Criag W. Evaluation of an ecological program to reduce bullying in schools. *Can J Counsel* 2002; **36**: 281–296.

83. Sanchez E, Robertson T, Lewis C *et al*. Preventing bullying and sexual harassment in elementary schools: the Expect Respect model. In: Geffner R, Loring M, Young C. (eds) *Bullying Behavior: Current Issues, Research, and Interventions*, Vol 2. New York, NY: Haworth Maltreatment & Trauma Press, 2001; 157–180.

84. Twemlow SW, Fonagy P, Sacco FC *et al*. Creating a peaceful school learning environment: a controlled study of an elementary school intervention to reduce violence. *Am J Psychiatry* 2001; **158**: 808–810.

85. Baldry AC, Farrington DP. Evaluation of an intervention program for the reduction of bullying and victimization in school. *Aggressive Behav* 2004; **30**: 1–15.

86. Boulton MJ, Flemington I. The effects of a short video intervention on secondary school pupils' involvement in definitions of and attitudes towards bullying. *School Psychol Int* 1996; **17**: 331–345.

87. Warden D, Moran E, Gillies J, Mayes G, Macleod L. An evaluation of a children's safety training programme. *Educ Psychol* 1997; **17**: 433–449.

88. Rican P, Ondrova K, Svatos J. The effect of a short, intensive intervention upon bullying in four classes in a Czech town. *Ann NY Acad Sci* 1996; **774**: 399–400.

89. Teglasi H, Rothman L. STORIES: a classroom-based program to reduce aggressive behavior. *J School Psychol* 2001; **39**: 71–94.

90. DeRosier ME. Building relationships and combating bullying: effectiveness of a school-based social skills group intervention. *J Clin Child Adolesc Psychol* 2004; **33**: 196–201.

91. Fast J, Fanelli F, Salen L. How becoming mediators affects aggressive students. *Child Schools* 2003; **25**: 161–171.

92. Meyer N, Lesch E. An analysis of the limitations of a behavioral programme for bullying boys from a subeconomic environment. *South Afr J Child Adolesc Mental Health* 2000; **12**: 59–69.

93. Tierney T, Dowd R. The use of social skills groups to support girls with emotional difficulties in secondary schools. *Support Learn* 2000; **15**: 82–85.

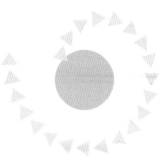

Index

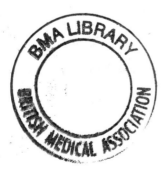